Learn Eyelash & Eyebrow Extensions-

Plus false and party eyelash applications.
With step by step instructions.

Complies with Beauty Therapy Code:- SIBBFAS302A
Provide lash and brow treatments updated and equivalent to
WRBFS305B Assessment Requirements
 for SHBBMUP001 Apply Eyelash Extensions 2018

~~~~~~**~~~~~

Author Robyn Ji. Smith

Revised 13th June 2010
31st October 2015
April 2019
August 2023
ISBN: 978-0-9945693-6-3

BISAC: Education / Training & Certification
Size 6x9" Full Colour on White paper

Copyright Page

INDEX

Index 1

Appointment questions 4

Patch Test 5

Tray Setup 7

Procedure. - Eyelash Extensions 9

Eyelash Material 13

Eyelash shapes. 18

Answers for clients 25

Technicians duty of care 30

Procedure Explained In More Detail. 33

Eyelash Protocol sheet 47

The Most Important Steps 51

The Amount of Glue 54

Eyelash Glue 60

Beauty Slant Position 65

Natural Eye Cleansing Solution: 66

Removing Eyelash Extensions 68

Test 1 Eyelash Extensions 73

How to submit your exams 74

Forms for client 75

Eye Anatomy 80

The basic processes of cell growth are: 82

The Anatomy of the Skin Around the Eyes 84

Eye diseases 86

Eyelash Transplants 92

Eyelash Growth Cycle. 93

Maintaining Healthy Skin Around the Eyes 96

Eye Treatment 97

Train Your Client Brochure. 99

Aftercare dos and don'ts 99

Eyes Draw Creams In 104

Aromatherapy Skincare 106

Making Skin Care 107

Aromatherapy Eye Exfoliate 115

Aromatherapy Do's and Don'ts: 118

To reduce, puffy eyes. 119

Aromatherapy Safe Oils 120

Aromatherapy Contra-indications 125

Important Factors 126

Test Three 130

Advertise Your Service. 131

Test Four 132

Test Aftercare Instructions 132

Test Five 135

Test Six Written exam 135

Party Lashes 139

Eyelash Education 142

HOW TO KEEP YOURSELF SAFE FROM LASH ADHESIVES 147

Applying Glue to Strip Lashes 148

Party Lashes, Verses Grafted Lashes. 151

Watch You Tube Video 152

A Typical Eyelash Extension Kit 154

Health and safety 157

Care more so the client sings your praises.

Dear Student.. 158

Certificate Course 161

Required Skills And Knowledge 162

Dear home user, ... 163

Eyebrow extensions Info 1

Tinting the Eyebrows: 11

Other books by 14

Beauty school Books 14

The index is a very helpful place to find what you need to know right now. However, I feel it is best to settle back with a cuppa away from the maddening crowd, and read the entire manual first But remember you will only gain great skills by practicing each explanation.

APPOINTMENT QUESTIONS

Also read "Appointment Instruction" page 25

1. At the appointment setting time - ask appropriate question.
2. Have you had eyelash extensions applied before?
3. If it is their first set they will need to have a patch test the day or at least week before. Explain the importance of a patch test.
4. Have they ever had an eye disorder – Stye, dry eyes, do your eyes water, do you cry easily?
5. Ask for their name and telephone number plus their email address.
6. Ask if they can send you those details so you can check what you have written down is correct.
7. Explain you will be sending client information form for them to fill in and the "Eyelash Preparation Form" If they have any questions they should call you.

PREPARATION FOR EYELASH EXTENSIONS

1. Check that the client form has been -filled in correctly.
2. Check the client is a suitable candidate?
3. Check eyes are healthy and the clients eyes do not water easily.
4. Decide what shape eyelashes the client needs for her face shape. However, the client might have a definite idea about the thickness and shape she/he wants. You are the professional and

Care more so the client sings your praises.

should give guidance, being careful not to force your opinion on them.

5. Add the advice you gave to the client form and have them sign that they have requested lashes too long for their skin or natural lash type. This explanation will be different for each client. Most client will heed to your advice, if it has been given in an informative way.
6. Do the patch test on new client.
7. Set out the eyelash mapping chart and have them approve the mapping chart.
8. Prepare the client
9. Clean their eyelashes and begin the procedure.
10. Take before and after photos and add to their file.

PATCH TEST

1. Conduct a full consultation and fill in all relevant forms.
2. Perform a patch test on all new clients.
3. Ask them to come with a clean face and no eye makeup.
4. Shine a torch in her eyes to check that her eyes do not water easily and for diseases.
5. Check on their form or ask them do their eyes water.
6. Also check for eye mites with your magnifying glasses.
7. Apply **one** lash to each eye. Do so as thought you are conducting a full procedure.
8. Use different glue on each eye.
9. Make notes on which glue was put on each eye.
10. You can do this any time but at least 24 hours before the applications.

However, if the client has stressed some makeup causes a reaction. **DO NOT DO THE PATCH TEST ON THEIR EYES**. Place one type of glue behind her left ear and another type behind her right ear. Also place the eyelash tape behind her ear a few inches away from her glue. Write notes on her file what glue went behind each ear. When testing glue sensitivity behind the ear you do not need to add an eyelash extension.

Clean all the tools you are going to use and place them in a location easy to reach. I like my mobile trolley to be close to my right hip.

I recommend watching this video
https://www.youtube.com/watch?v=2XwnJFM6iP0

MAGNIFYING GLASSES ARE A MUST NO MATTER HOW GOOD YOUR EYESIGHT IS.

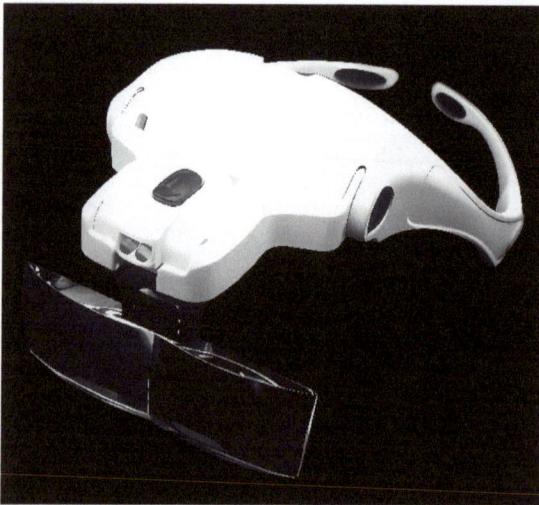

TRAY SETUP

1. Cleanser
2. Toner
3. Eyelash cleaner
4. Primer (Depends on glue type)
5. Contact lens case and liquid.
6. Face cloth
7. Bowl and towel
8. Kidney bowl
9. Saline or eye cleanser to flash the eyes.
10. Kidney shaped bowl
11. Cotton wool pads
12. Hand towels must be white so they can be disinfected after each use.
13. 2 Good quality rubber sponges to clean around eyes
14. Eye Tape
15. Protection pads
16. Tooth picks
17. Premium eyelash 15mm or .20mm diameters, in lengths of 8 mm /10mm/12mm /14mm
18. Pad to sit eyelashes on
19. Micro buds
20. Cotton buds
21. Glue (black sensitive) 1 bottle 10 ml,
22. Glass or jade plate to put glue on
23. Glue Remover 1
24. Extension /volume -up Mascara *(optional)*
25. Three sets of tweezers. Two off curved type. Two off Straight type.
26. Mini hand held mirror
27. Hand Towel
28. Mini scissors

29. Rubber air-blower
30. 2 sets of false eyelashes. To give client an idea of how their lashes will look.
31. Medical adhesive tape
32. Pads to protect bottom lashes and skin
33. Comb-brush for eyelash
34. 1 Eyelash curler (use a heat source to straighten eyelashes)
35. 2 Eyelash wands
36. Paper towel (white)
37. Tissues
38. Magnifying glasses. *Buy the very best.*
39. Torch
40. Head band for client
41. Alcohol wipes to clean tweezers during procedure.

Note: The eyelash curling wand can also be used a straightening iron. Place on the upper lash on the top of the lashes. Place a comb at the base or a brush. Press

the wand and the comb together and pull straight out. This is only required if they have excessive curl in their natural lashes.

PROCEDURE. - EYELASH EXTENSIONS

For a new client a patch test should be performed at least 24 hours prior. At consultation time shine a torch in their eyes. Just wave over each eye do not hold torch directly into the eye. If their eyes water they are not a candidate for eyelash extensions. If the patch test went well and the torch did not cause their eyes to water then you can proceed. Providing they have no eye diseases.

1. Put on a pair of gloves.
2. Conduct a thorough eye exam.
3. Use your magnifying glasses and a tooth pick to separate the lashes while viewing the root area. If the client has no visible signs of eye diseases you can proceed.
4. Have a thin and a thick set of false eyelashes to show client how her lashes will look. If she has very thick dark lashes hold the thick false lashes with tweezes to her eyelid. If she has thin natural lashes hold the thin strip of false lashes to her eyelid.
5. Show her the eyelash shape diagram.
6. Talk to her about her face shape and suggest the style of the lash shape.
7. Check if your client is using contact lens. If she is, she will need to remove them and place in the contact case.
8. Remove and dispose of gloves.
9. Fill in all forms.
10. Set up tray and place on mobile trolley
11. Place paper towel sheet on your beauty bed and make the client comfortable.
12. Apply a head band to hold her hair back.

13. Make sure you have enough light.
14. Your client must be in a comfortable position lying on cosmetic bed.
15. Start out with a clean, fresh face and very clean and dry eyelashes.
16. **Important:** Do not curl eyelashes before applying extension. This is only required when clients eyelashes are extremely straight.
17. The straighter eyelashes are, the easier they will bond with the glue. Some clients have frizzy lashes that need a warm wand to straighten before the graft application. Warm the wand and use the eyelash comb followed by the wand in an outward stroke not in a curling motion.
18. Determine how you are going to place your lashes, choose the sizes of the lashes you going to use and locate near you. Place them on a pad on her shoulder is a manageable place to sit them. Or use an eyelash bracelet.
19. This may be the time to wash your hands and put on fresh gloves.
20. Comb and brush her natural lashes well.
21. Place the sticky tape to the bottom lashes. There must be no visible signs of the bottom lashes.
22. Now comb her top lashes again.
23. Place a half moon shaped pad over the bottom lashes and under her top lashes.
24. Add tape to the eyelids in both corners of the lids to pull the lid corners up. I also add tape across the eyelids just above the top of the upper lash root area...
25. Separate the top lashes and have one lash between the straight pair of tweezers.
26. The natural lash should be in the **telogen stage** of growth.

27. Pick up one extension lash with tweezes be sure the thick end is at the bottom of the tweezers.
28. Carefully dip the thick end in glue.
29. Rock the glue lash end back and forth on the glass pad or jade plate pad to remove excess glue.
30. Apply to the lash you have chosen. Run the glue end up the natural lash then position the extension lash about 2-3 mm away from the natural lash base..
31. Use the tooth pick or another set of tweezers to position the extension lash running upward with the natural lash. Extension lashes are heavier then natural lashes and often want to fall to the side. Use tooth picks to align the natural and extension lash together as a united pair.
32. Blow the glue with the air pump.
33. When applying do a few lashes on each eye.
34. Use the blower often to soothe here eyes and dry the glue.
35. Depending on the lash mapping that has been agreed to apply lash extensions.
36. After applying a few lashes to each eye get up move to the front of the client and use a tooth pick to roll the underside of the lashes up. Check that they are not sticking to the bottom lash tape and that the lash glue is not sticking to the lash next to the lash you have extended. You can also use a dental mirror to check the underside of the lashes.
37. Apply the required amount of 25 to 30 lashes. To each eye.
38. As you add a lash extension- check that there is no pooling of glue and that the glue is a few millimetres away from the lid/skin and above the lash root.
39. Blow the lashes with the pump style blower.
40. As you work on each lash be confident, they have not attached to the lashes each side of the new lash extension. Use tweezers and tooth picks to separate

the new lash. Hold for a few seconds and blow with the hand pump blower.

41. When you have completed both sides blow each eye with the hand pump blower.
42. **Wait for 5 to 10 minutes**. Check that the client is comfortable. During this time you could gentle massage her brow and forehead area.
43. Gently comb the lashes one eye at a time.
44. Rinse her eyes with the saline mix.
45. Place mild eye drops in her eyes.
46. Check her eyes after asking her to blink several times.
47. Should the client want more lashes you can then begin your second layer.
48. Be sure to place a cold pack on her eyes.
49. After she has checked in the mirror and has confirmed she is happy, you can remove the pads under her eyes.
50. Clean the eye area with saline
51. Go through the aftercare procedure with her.
52. Give her a warm drink and check she is stable after getting up off the bed.

The size of extensions will depend on the shape and length the client wants.

Although her eyes need a good rinse be certain not to get the glue wet. I usually hold a cloth on her top lashes as I rinse her eyes. Place her head to the side. Use a kidney bowl pressed to her face to catch the saline.

If you need to remove old lash extensions first see my section on removing eyelash extensions.

New extensions **should not** be applied the same day as you remove old extensions. You need to explain this at the appointment setting time. Do not wait until they have arrived. They may have a special event to go to.

The tray setup and the procedure instructions are here as counsel but naturally you are not ready to perform your first set of lashes. You need to study many things first and practice this art many times before you practice on a human.

EYELASH MATERIAL

Silk: Silk lashes are softer and slightly glossy. Faux Mink: These are finer than silk, so it's necessary to apply a few more lashes. The extra fluff is nice for special occasions.

Mink Lashes: Made from real mink fur, mink lashes provide a very realistic lash that most closely resembles natural eyelashes.

Mink and Silk lashes are very light Mink lashes do not hold their curl as well as other types of lashes and you may need to curl them between salon visits.

Synthetic material: Most extensions fall in this category and are made from a plastic fibre called PBT (Polybutylene Terephthalate).

Lash lengths vary from as short as six millimetres to an impressive 17 millimetres. The length you choose depends on the look and comfortability that you're going for. Synthetic materials are the most requested fibres for eyelash extensions because they are affordable, don't cause harm to animals, and are easy to use. Silk lash extensions come in second place because of their lightweight and comfortability.

LASH SHAPES & THICKNESS OUTLINE

Synthetic Lashes come in
Types: "J" – "C" – "D"
Thickness: 0,07 mm
Length: 8 mm. – 9 mm. – 10 mm. – 11 mm. – 13 mm.– 14
Suppliers will list like this
Types: "J" – "C" – "D"

Thickness:
0,10 mm. – 0,15 mm. – 0,20 mm. – 0,25 mm.
Length:
7 mm. – 9 mm. – 11 mm. – 13 mm. – 15 mm.

Synthetic & Mink Lashes
Types: " C" and "D "
Thickness: 0,15 mm. – 0,20 mm.
Length: 8 mm. – 10 mm. – 12 mm. – 14 mm.

3D Mink lashes
Types: "J" – "C" – "D"
Thickness: 0,07 mm
Length: 8 mm. – 9 mm. – 10 mm. – 11 mm. – 13 mm.– 14 mm.
Check with your supplier to confirm this information.

EYELASH SIZES: & CURL TYPES

You will need to view the suppliers' charts. I feel the standard ""C" curl to be the best. 07 is my favourite diameter. You will need all lengths in stock. Because it will depend on the height of the clients face what lengths you use. The distance between the open eyelid and their eyebrow, plays a major role.

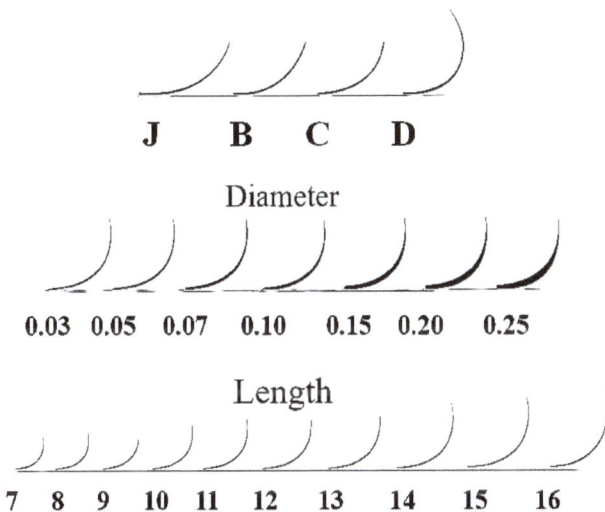

| J | B | C | D |

Diameter

0.03 0.05 0.07 0.10 0.15 0.20 0.25

Length

7 8 9 10 11 12 13 14 15 16

Pots of lashes are the cheapest way to buy lashes. There is one size per pot. The most used sizes are 8 mm, 10 mm and 12 mm. The only issues I have found are there are sometimes some odd shaped lashes and some lashes are half a lash. You get a great number of lashes per jar, so that did not bother me. You sprinkle the lashes onto a pad.

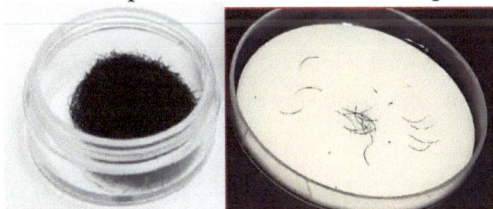

This is a slightly slower method because you sprinkle the lashes on a pad and they are all sitting in different directions. You pick a lash up then you have to use the other set of tweezers to put the lash in the tweezers the way you need them to sit and then swop hands. That is time consuming.

As pictured below you can purchase them in strips. They come several ways. One strip can have all of one size or some strips can be purchased as a multi strip with about two rows of each different size.
When buying strips pay the extra money and buy them locally. They can often be moisture damaged and when they are damages from moisture, **they are a nightmare to work** with. I purchased a large quantity from Beauty Expo once, off an Asian stand. Not one strip was usable. They were hard to remove from the strip and when I did manage to get a lash off the strip, each lash had paper attached to the end.

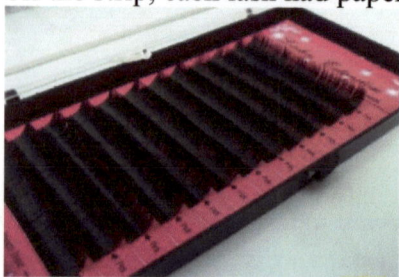

However, if you can get fresh lashes from a reputable supplier, they are the best to use.
They are a perfect shape and thickness. They are easy and quick to use. But only when they are in an individual sealed box per strip.
It is best to buy them in one size per strip and have an application board that you apply the three sizes you need onto the board.
Also see my other suggestions below in the YouTude video.

Care more so the client sings your praises.

http://www.youtube.com/watch?v=Z5LQimFojKI

In this video the therapist positions the lash with the tweezers that she applied the lash with. Never ever allow your tweezers to come in contact with the glue. This will cause lots of problems. The main problem will be the tweezers will glue together and with glue on the tweezers other natural lashes may stick to the tweezers. When she applies the second lash, she uses the correct tool to position the lash.

Never wipe the glue onto the clients eye pad. Have a small glass pad sitting near the client's neck or on her chest. I use a plastic wrap under the eye not these white pads. They pull too much on the sensitive skin around the eyes. They are fine if you cut them in half. She also puts the glue too close to the skin.

With that said, for your education purposes I would like to add, it is a nerve-racking experience being on video while you are working. Unlike movie makers that have a big budget to produce a movie with lots of reruns these therapist get one shot.

EYELASH SHAPES.

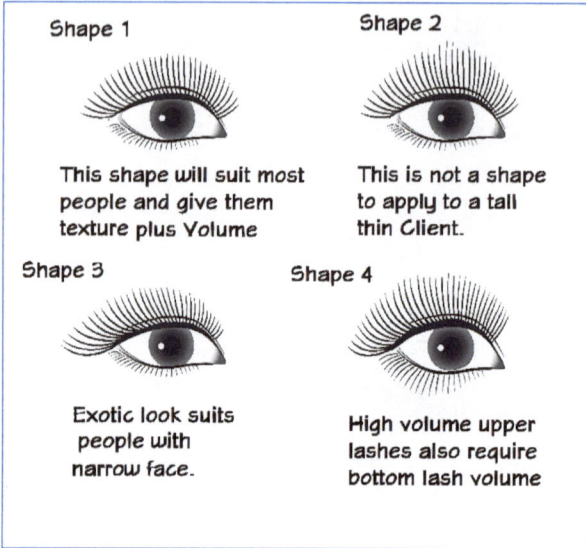

Shape 1

This shape will suit most people and give them texture plus Volume

Shape 2

This is not a shape to apply to a tall thin Client.

Shape 3

Exotic look suits people with narrow face.

Shape 4

High volume upper lashes also require bottom lash volume

Shape 1 should not be applied to a client with a moon shape face.

Shape 2 should not be applied to a client with a long face.

Shape 2 should not be applied to a client that is tall and thin.

Shape 2 should not be applied to a client with a high/large forehead.

Shape 3 suits all clients. However - if they have eyes set with a large space between the eyes add thicker style lashes to the middle and a few thicker lashes scattered between the thinner lashes. If you have used thick lashes use some finer thickness of lashes scattered along the eye lid between the tick lashes.

Shape 4 is best suited to larger framed women or women with strong facial features.

Shape 2 and 4 are ideal for mature aged people. High lashes in the middle open the eye more.

Care more so the client sings your praises.

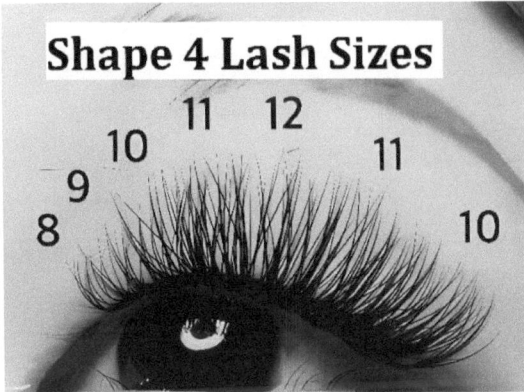

Shape 4 Lash Sizes

It is best to map out where you are going to place the different size and the thickness of each lash.

EXTENSION /VOLUME   LASHES

Can be used sparingly but never as a full set of lashes. They are too heavy even for thick and strong natural lashes. They are small bunches of lashes. Place single lashes between the extension /volume   lashes.

Remember less is best. 20 to 30 lashes spaced evenly across their natural eyelash is plenty. The thickness of the extension lash will depend on their natural lash thickness.

Not all of their natural lashes will be in the correct growth stage to attach an extension lash too.

Note: For a mature aged person it is better that the lashes are longer in the middle. This will make the eyes more wide open.

The shorter the lashes are in the inner corner near the nose the more open your client eyes will look. Too long in that position creates an aged tired look.

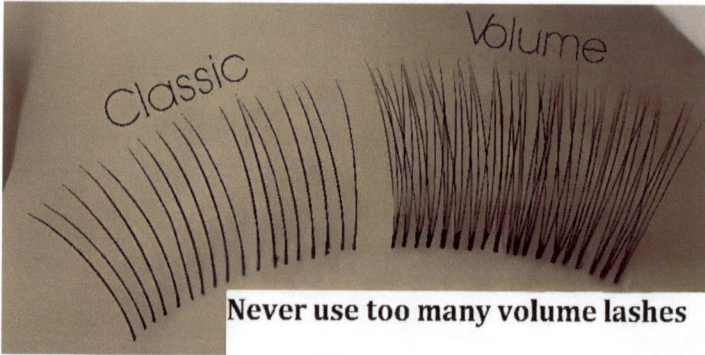

Never use too many volume lashes

It is impossible to cover all you need to know about eyelash thickness and shapes to suit a face type and shape. There is so much to consider.

The texture of the clients skin, the colour and tone of their skin, their hair style and colour, their eyebrow shape and colour and an endless amount of other issues. All this will become second nature after you have practiced on an orange and later on friends and family.

I hope to do more within the next two years in my book called "**Create Eyebrows To Suit Face Shapes.**" This book is in infancy as I need at least six months to gather photos. Then another twelve months to put the information together. However, it is available on Amazon and will assist you with face shapes. But expect a better book next year.

In the mean time think about this:-.

Shape 3 in the above diagram is called the exotic look and is also known as Almond shaped eyes. The almond shape lashes are very attractive and any eye shape will flutter up quite nicely with lashes that are longer at the outer edge that create an almond shape. It is your safety shape, because it looks good on all clients.

Care more so the client sings your praises.

Never put very thick lashes on a client with tiny features and fine hair.

Never put thin fine lashes on a client that has dark complexion. thick hair and thick black natural lashes. Spend at least one hour every night for the next five weeks or so researching before and after shots of eyelash extensions on the internet and start forming your own opinions.

This is why it pays to have lots of photos to show the client. You will also be well advised to buy packets of false eyelashes of all different thicknesses and extension /volume to hold on one of the clients eyes.

The concluding resolution must always be the client choice. However, you should be educated well enough to advise him/her. A clever adviser will always allow the end decision to be that of the one being advised.

PRACTICE LASHES TO BUY

Buy some false eyelashes to experiment with. Hold them on family members and friends. Take note on how the different thickness, lengths and shapes suit different people.

When you hold one row of fine false lashes on a client that needs thick lashes you will soon realize that this client needs thick mink lashes. When you hold thick black false lashes on a client of a small build with fine hair and thin eyebrows you will be quick to notice how silly she looks.

Eyelash Grafting and Party Lashes

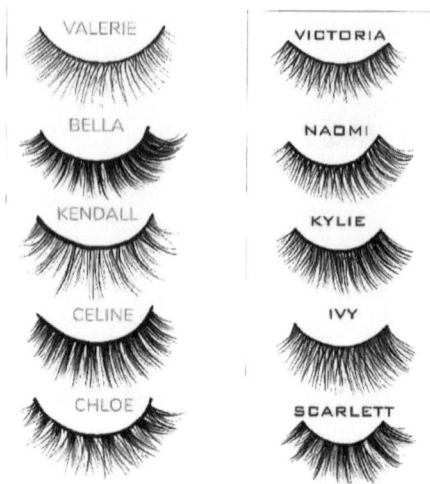

VALERIE · VICTORIA · BELLA · NAOMI · KENDALL · KYLIE · CELINE · IVY · CHLOE · SCARLETT

For these reasons you need to purchase many sets of false lashes and a variety of extension lashes.

WHAT YOU'LL NEED FOR LASH MAPPING:

1. Eyeliner or pencil. This is for mapping on the skin first.
2. Gel pads. These are placed over the lower lashes while you work.
3. A coloured pen. This is for marking on the gel pad - you want a colour that will contrast with the eyelashes - red is a good choice. We recommend avoiding black pen if you can as your markings will be harder to spot, but if it's all you have, place your markers further away from the lashes.

For Lash extensions. You'll need various lengths, a few curls types, a few different thicknesses', single lashes and bunches of lashes.

APPOINTMENT INSTRUCTIONS

When a client or prospective client makes that first call to enquire about eyelash extensions, do not just quote prices. If you do not have time to explain the different types of lashes ask if you can call her back and what would be the best time.

If you are in the middle of a procedure, tell the new client. Give them an appointment time but explain you will require their email address for the before care sheet and price list. Prices should be according to style and thickness. The client may simply want to book in and that is great. Try never to give a flat price over the phone.

Take her name, telephone number and her email address and make the appointment, no matter how busy you are you need her email and telephone number.

As soon as possible send her an email and a text message to her mobile. You could, while you are on the telephone ask her if she could text her email and phone number to your mobile. Land lines are great but mobiles are more user friendly and every salon should have a mobile phone as well as a land line.

However, still take her details then ask her to confirm them via text. Have a standard message that you send to all clients set up on your mobile phone. If the client has called your landline while on the phone send her the standard message this way she can confirm she has received your message while you are still talking to her. Your standard message could say - " Hi this is Sally from Beauty by Sally 105 Gold Coast Hwy Burleigh Heads. Later today I will send you some forms. Thank you for your time and I look forward to meeting you. Sally."

If she is unsure of the service, you need to talk her through her options and explain the price range and why there is a range of options.

1. Does the client want a natural look or a dramatic look?
2. How long does she want to have the lashes for?
3. Is it just for a special occasion or is it going to be an ongoing look?

You need to explain the different between: -

1. A few bunches of lashes at the outer corner.
2. False lashes for special occasions
3. The standard 25 grafted lashes to each eye for the natural look and 30 or more lashes for a more dramatic look and volume lashes.
4. Explain the growth stages of eyelashes and that you as a professional charge more for clients that want to have lashes on long term, as you need to find the eyelashes that are in Talogen growth stage. But it is better to explain this after you have sent her a brief email explaining the growth stage of eyelashes.
5. If the client has not had lash extensions before explain she will be required to have a patch test done and how important that is.

The more informative you are the more professional you will sound. Yet you do not want to bombard her with needless information.

It is important to send her via text or email - her preparation notes. This lets her know all the things she should do before her appointment.

Care more so the client sings your praises.

All too often you tell them not to wear mascara and they arrive with very thick layers of mascara. That is not her fault it is yours. No one remembers all that they hear and most clients do not study beauty therapy and do not understand the importance of your requests. Lashes do not last as long when they come to the salon with eyes that need a good clean.

Send her these two diagrams with the notes on how to prepare her lashes for the treatment. Sell her on your professionalism. Do not bombard her with information. Wet her appetite, so she feels safe and realizes why she needs to come with mascara free and clean eyelashes. Your professional manner will give her a reason to pay you more than others charge.

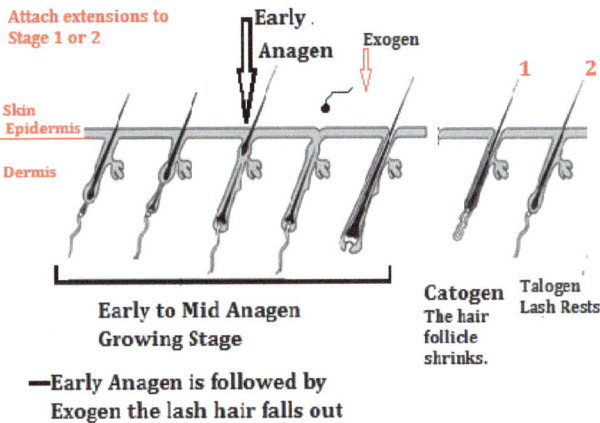

Attach extensions to Stage 1 or 2

Early Anagen

Exogen

Skin Epidermis

Dermis

1 2

Early to Mid Anagen
Growing Stage

Catogen
The hair follicle shrinks.

Talogen
Lash Rests

—Early Anagen is followed by Exogen the lash hair falls out

ANSWERS FOR CLIENTS

Arm yourself with answers to their questions.
These are some of the questions I have found clients ask and an idea on how to answer those questions.

Eyelash Grafting and Party Lashes

WHAT ARE EYELASH EXTENSIONS?

Eyelash extensions are a popular new service that lengthens
and thickens your own natural eyelashes. Lash extensions are
single strands of synthetic eyelashes that are curved to
replicate a natural eyelash.

They are applied to each individual natural eyelash one by
one for a natural, beautiful and luscious look.

Eyelash extensions are perfect for both, day to day wear or a
special occasion.

False lashes are a row of lashes that sit on your natural
lashes. They are on a small thin string and are not designed to
last as long as grafted lashes. Eyelash extensions have been
around since the time of Cleopatra as far as we know.
However, today's methods are far superior.

CAN I HAVE VERY THICK LASHES

We will view your eyelash type under our magnifier and
advise you at the time of your consultation. Extension
/volume   lashes are tiny bunches of lashes. Due to their extra
weight they are not suitable for all clients. People with fine
skin are usually advised not to have them. They can appear
fake. They also age the face in photos.

IF I DON'T LIKE THEM CAN I TAKE THEM OFF.

Yes, we can take them off or advise you how to take them
off. However, if we have done our job properly then it will
not be easy. The bonding agent is very strong. You will also
lose some of your natural lashes in the process. At the time of
your consultation we will hold a few different types of false
lashes on our eyes. You can then choose the shape and

Care more so the client sings your praises.

thickness you like. Should you not like the look - you are free to cancel your appointment. The cancelation fee is just $25.

WHAT HAPPENS IF I DEVELOP AN ALLERGY?

Call us immediately and we will remove the lashes for you. This is providing you have not developed blisters that have burst and are bleeding. We do **not** have a surgically sterile room. "Anyone who experiences an infection, any inflammation, an allergic reaction or a noticeable loss of natural eyelashes should see an ophthalmologist immediately." However, this is rear and we will conduct a patch teat first to alleviate this problem.

You can remove them with olive oil and an eyelash comb. The faster you attend to the removal process the better. Start with a ice pack to soothe the eyes.

Chamomile oil is the best essential oil healer for your eyelids. Add one drop of Chamomile essential oil to three tablespoons of olive oil.
Use a mascara shaped brush, dip in the olive oil mix and apply to the Lashes. Allergies are rear and we always perform a patch test for new clients.

HOW LONG DO LASH EXTENSIONS LAST?

We provide a guide sheet on how to care for your lashes. Properly applied extensions should last as long as your natural lash life cycle. That is anywhere from 3-10 weeks, depending on the individual. Of course rubbing, crying or pulling will make them shed quicker. Aftercare is the key to longevity. An infill every 2-3 weeks is recommended.

Eyelash Grafting and Party Lashes

We here at *(Name Your Salon)* pride ourselves in finding natural lashes that are in the talogen stage of growth. That guarantees a better chance of longer lasting lashes. It also guarantees - less damage to the natural lash regeneration process.

HOW OFTEN SHOULD I GET TOUCH-UPS?

We recommend getting a touch up every 2 to 4 weeks. If you wait too long your eyelash extensions will fall out. Your natural eyelashes fall off every 25 - 60 days due to the natural growth cycle and are naturally replaced with the growth of a new eyelash.

Other factors such as exposure to steam or touching your eyes a lot may cause the extensions to fall sooner. A touch up is needed to fill in any lashes that have fallen. Touch ups average about 45 minutes.

CAN I SWIM, SHOWER, EXERCISE, OR VISIT A SPA WHILE WEARING EYELASH EXTENSIONS?

The bonding agent we use is waterproof. Therefore, you can shower, swim, exercise. Special care is required. Yet overall maintenance is low. It is advisable **not** to wash your eye area for about 5-10 hours after the application.

Try not to cry as tears contain salty liquids. Our new, industry leading eyelash extensions adhesive no longer requires the 12 - 24 hours. We will give you our complete aftercare procedures. However we may need to use a different type of glue if you have sensitive skin and it takes up to 12 hours to set.

HOW LONG WILL IT TAKE TO APPLY EYELASH EXTENSIONS AND HOW IS IT DONE?

The application process for lash extensions normally takes anywhere from 45 min. - 1.5 hours. You will lay comfortably on a massage or facial bed with your eyes closed. The eyelash professional will then apply an under eye gel pad to cover your lower lashes. Check eyelash health and prepare you. Then the extensions will be applied to each individual eyelash on a hair by hair basis. It is important that we do not attach them to baby lashes. Our therapist takes pride in attaching them to a telogen stage of growth lash. Then your infill treatments will take 30-45 minutes.

WHAT SHOULD I DO TO PREPARE FOR THE PROCEDURE?

Please refrain from applying eye makeup 48 hours prior to coming in for the procedure. You eyelashes should be free of enhancers such as shadows and mascara. A good exfoliate and cleaning process will be attached to your welcome email.

The extensions are connected with glue and therefore any debris may shorten the lifecycle of the extensions and cause them to fall off earlier.

In case makeup application is inevitable for you, we do have makeup remover and face wash available at our salon for your convenience. We also offer a full cleanse service for a small fee of *(put a price here)*.

We recommend that you remove your contact lenses prior to receiving the procedure. Your eyes will be closed while receiving your extensions and your contact lens may cause eye dryness. Removing contacts will remarkably increase your comfort level. We have a contact lens disposable case here for your lens. There is a small charge or you may bring your own case. We will email you the prep sheet.

TECHNICIANS DUTY OF CARE

You have a duty of care to all people at all times. Therefore, they need to receive a before Eyelash Grafting Care Sheet. It should contain these instructions.

1. Ask client to clean their eyelashes with olive oil one-two days before the procedure and thoroughly remove all dry skin around their eyes. They could use a tiny pinch of corn flower mixed with the olive oil.
2. To remove the oil mix they first use soft tissues or cotton wool pads.
3. Next with eyes closed massage in a mild cleansing lotion or baby shampoo, be very gentle.

4. Slash water on the eyes many times.
5. Pat dry.
6. Then with a warm face cloth, press the eyes.
7. Follow by pressing the eyes with a cold cloth.
8. Ask the client not to wear eye makeup nor mascara one –two days prior to the treatment.
9. If the client has not performed the above procedure you will need to do a complete cleanse of the eye

area. Next use a warm compress several times. This will ensure there is no oil residue.

10. Then apply an ice pack for five minutes to their closed eyes to close the skin pores.

11. **In their preparation sheet add a small explanation of why it is important <u>not</u> to wear mascara for one to two days prior to treatment. Cleaning the lashes methodically on the same day as the extensions decreases the ability for the glue and their natural lashes to bond.**

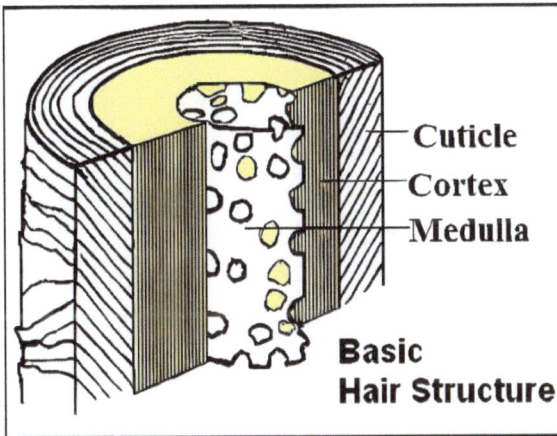

Cuticle
Cortex
Medulla

Basic Hair Structure

A. It is important for them to understand that lashes have a core and cells. These cells accumulate tiny particles of debris. The Cuticle is like tiny fish scales and that is where oil gets trapped. Cleaning products also get stuck under the scales. This should also help them to understand the importance of brushing their lashes.

B. If the client has not cleaned her eyes well before the treatment, she **must sign a disclaimer** stating you cannot guarantee the bond.

C. As I have explained before you will need to clean their face and eyelashes before applying extensions. You should charge for this extra service. They must also sign a disclaimer - that states the glue may not bond as well as it would have if they had done their eye cleansing 48 hours ago. Then left their eyes without makeup and mascara during the 48 hour period.

D. Explain that they should not remove the lashes themself with eyelash removing products. They have strong chemicals that may harm their eyes.

PROCEDURE EXPLAINED IN MORE DETAIL.

1. Fill in all forms
2. Be sure you have checked with the client as to how long she wants the lashes. Show her some photos of different lengths.
3. Be sure you have checked her face shape and know the correct style and shape of the lashes for the client. Refer to book "Eyebrow Shaping & Tinting" In section covering face shapes.
4. Check eyes for diseases and dirt.
5. Do the patch test 24 hours before the procedure.
6. Lay the client on a comfortable bed that has been lowered. Their eyes should be level with your waist. This gives you an excellent view of their eyelid. Looking over the top of her eyes is the best view for extension application. Her head should be tilted back so you can see their natural lash line.
7. Never ever have the client sitting in a chair. In a Hairdressing salon you may have them at the shampoo basin with a pillow under their neck, providing you are standing on a step beside them and they are comfortable.
8. I strongly recommend you only sit client at a salon basin for false and party lash application. Never have them at the basin for eyelash grafting.
9. You need to be able to move around the client freely.
10. You must be at least 600 mm above their eyes.
11. It is unwise to trim the lashes after they are complete. The lashes have been manufactured to curve at 3 mm above the base. That is why they come in a range of sizes. and shapes. The manufacturers have gone to

great lengths to tapper the lashes at the tip and if you trim them they will look blunt and unnatural.

12. Place a few lashes on a smooth white makeup sponge.
13. Place the sponge on the bed near her head. You need a sponge for each of the different sizes.
14. When using the lashes that come in strips have them placed close to the clients head, on your wrist or on a strip holder.
15. Note: These types of lashes come in different ways. I like to buy the strips that have all the different size lashes on the one strip. I place the strip on either the client forehead or on the wrist of my **non** dominate hand. This is my left hand.

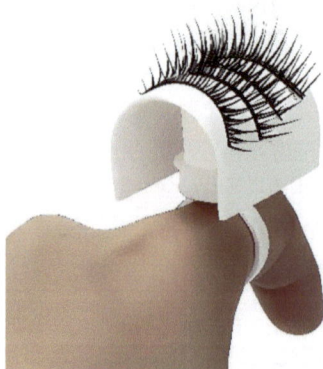

16. There are finger and wrist bands available on eBay.
17. The client must be made to feel comfortable. Do not ask questions that the client is able to answer with "Yes or No".
18. Ask the client to explain how comfortable or uncomfortable she is.
19. **Ash her - What would you like me to change?**
20. Example: Do you need this pillow under your knees moved up or down?
21. When you set up your tray have it very close to you.

22. Now clean the eye area with cleaning fluid. Use a cotton pad to apply and dry with clean cotton pads.
23. Next use the pump to blow the eye lashes dry.
24. The natural lashes must be completely cleaned and free of residue. Their natural lashes must be soft and exceptionally free of oil.
25. With the clients eyes open place a piece of glad wrap or masking tape under the upper lashes and over the bottom lashes.
26. Be sure the wrap does not touch their eyeball and that it completely covers the bottom lashes. You are covering the bottom lashes so you can protect them from glue and to prevent the top and bottom lashes sticking together.
27. My preferred method is 4 to 5 pieces of medical tape.
28. The aloe vera pads don't do a good enough job for me. They seem to slide.
29. However, to use plastic lunch wrap will stop eyes from watering. After placing it across the bottom lash area, gently roll back and tuck in the pierce covering the eyeball.
30. The next photo has the first two strips in place you then add two more strips or three more until the bottom lashes are well covered.
31. You can also buy lash pads.

32.

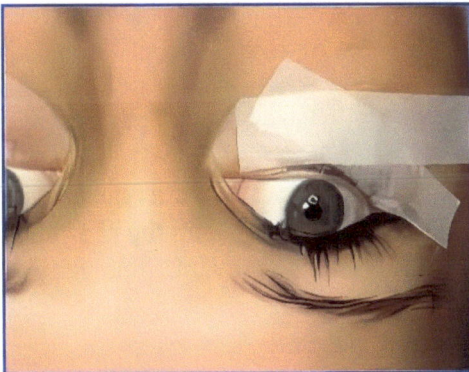

33. Use your magnifying glasses and be very certain that all the bottom lashes are completely covered and that you have no tape touching the inside of the eye and not sitting on the skin near the inside of the eyelash roots. Ask the client to blink and ask it her eye feels comfortable. Adjust if necessary. Then do the same to the other eye.

If the bottom lashes are not carefully held by the eye pad or tape during the lash process, the pop out ones can stick to the upper lashes. Therefore, when you have finished the set, remember to ask your clients to blink several times and make sure they don't feel the stickiness when they open their eyes. **Note** - in the above photo a third smaller pierce of tape - in the middle of were the tape crosses over, would be required to complete this action.

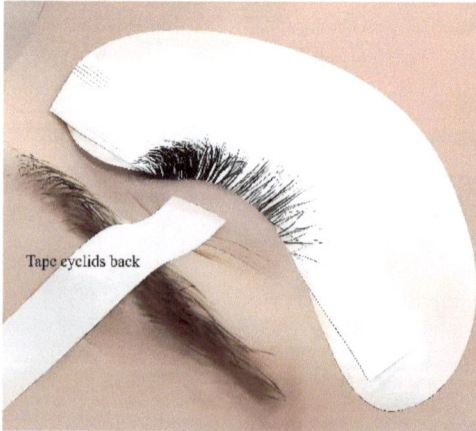

Tape eyelids back

34.

35. Tape the lids up with a pull towards the eyebrow area. This is of more importance when the client has dropping eye lids. It also prevents glue getting on

delicate eye skin. I like to put at least two tapes on in each end of the eyelid.

36. Then brush the upper lashes to be sure the upper lashes are sitting above the glad-wrap/ tape and the lower lashes are sitting under the glad wrap or tape.

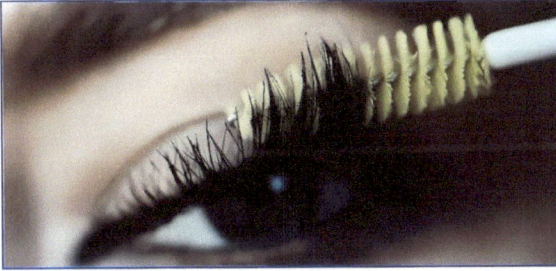

I like them to open their eyes during this brushing process.

37. Comb the upper lashes. Brush and comb the lashes well. I actually do not use cotton pads when applying lashes I use tape or plastic wrap to protect the skin. The cotton pad can stick to the glue.
38. Put a tiny amount of glue onto a piece of glass.
39. Place the glass close to the client on the bed or their chest. I do not like stretching over to the trolley.
40. Ask the client to close their eyes and keep them closed for the entire procedure.

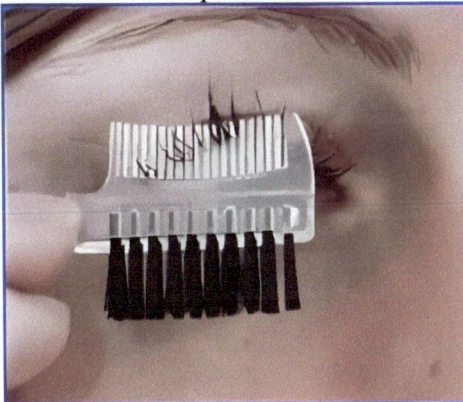

But I used a pad in this photo figure 1- so you could see me separating the lashes and to have just one lash in between my tweezers.

Figure 1 Lash Separation

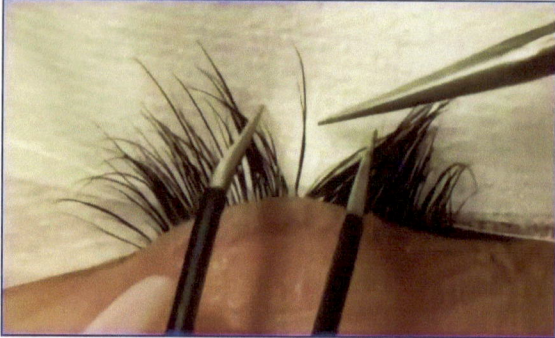

- Use your tweezers to push the lashes away from where you are going to apply the lash.

In the photo marked lash separation you can see the student has skilfully used her tweezers to keep the natural lashes each side of the lash extension placement.

One lash only must be between the open tweezers. Be certain that it is not a lash that already has a lash attached to it. **Use your hand pump to blow the lash dry before removing the tweezers that are holding the other lashes away.**

Pick up the thin end of the lash and dip the thicker end into some glue. Less is best. If you pick up too much glue wipe it off on the glass pad, or wipe excess glue on a thick eye pad that you have stuck to under the eyes. **The danger in using the pad to wipe off glue is you might touch it and spread elsewhere.**

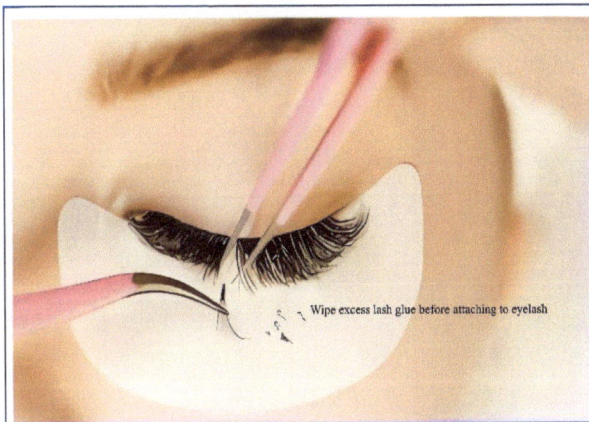

Wipe excess lash glue before attaching to eyelash

When you have dipped the eyelash in glue, brush the excess glue off the lash extension. Wipe the lash on the pad or the glass plate to remove some of the glue from the extension lash.

This decreases the amount of glue that is being put onto the natural lash. Too much glue and the clients will feel like they have heavy eyes.

Run the glue that is on the new lash up the length of the clients own lash. This will ensure the new lash sticks to the clients lash the full length of the clients natural lash. I like to use new tooth picks to set each lash in place.

Apply the extension lash to one of the client's lashes about **2 mm** up the lash. **Not at the root but close to the root. Never ever touch the skin with the glue**.

It is important to go from one eye to the other. Put two lashes at the outer corner of each eye. Then two lashes at the inner corner, of each eye. Then put two or three lashes in the center of each eye.

Infill each eye a few at a time. Place a few extensions on one eye then a few on the other eye. Never ever complete one eye first.

Do not rest your hand on the clients face. Use your little finger as a pivot.

Repeat this process until you have 25-30 lashes on both eyes. Should the client want more, you will need to charge them for the extra lashes, glue and your time.

When you have completed the lashes use a hand blower to dry the lashes. The clients love the feel of this gentle breeze on their eyes it is very soothing and dries the glue.

Do not use a hair dryer. The dryer below is also used for drying photos. Blow each lash before you release the tweezers that are holding the existing lashes apart. This is extremely important for many reasons.

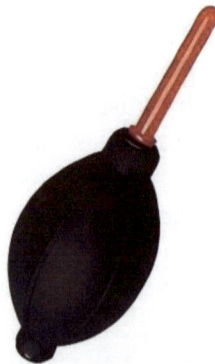

i.   A baby lash may stick to the new lash.
ii.   Humidity can cause new lash to bend.

iii.   Remember to keep a hygrometer in your lash studio, or find yourself a lash glue that performs well even in unstable room conditions.

iv.   The robust growth of Telogen phase (Baby) lashes can force the baby lash to push the extensions it's stuck to -to the side and leave you with a messy lash look.

v.   If glue attaches to a neighbouring lash it will cause a messy look. **Why?** Because all lashes are growing at different speeds.

Now separate all the lashes with two sets of tweezers. You can also use a tooth pick. I like to use tooth picks to separate the lashes and remove excess glue as I apply each lash.

Use your non dominate hand to hold the lash you intend to attach the extension to. With one set of tweezers hold the lashes each side away from the lash you have chosen to attach the extension too.

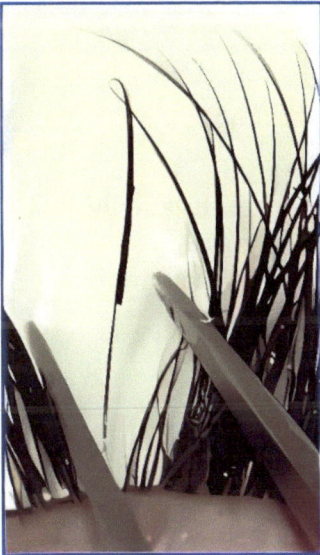

Pick up one extension, dip in glue, wipe excess off, attach to the natural lash 3 to 3 mm above root.

Place first lash on the outside near the temple. Go to the other eye and do the same.

Next place an extension in the middle of the eyelashes. Do the same on the other eye.

By doing one lash on each eye, you give the glue time to dry and avoid lashes sticking together. By alternating where each extension is placed also works well.

Use the had blower often.

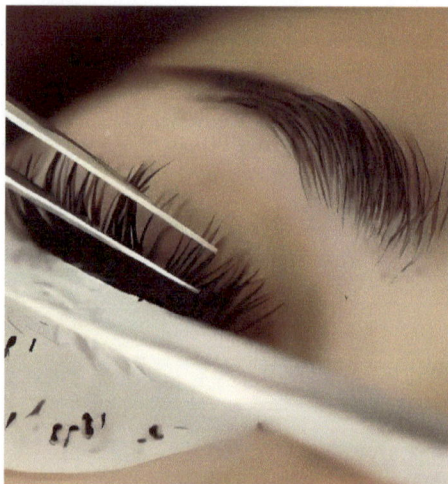

Check under the lashes to be sure it has not stuck to the pad under the eyes. Do this often during the procedure.

You can also view the client lashes with a dental mirror during the process.

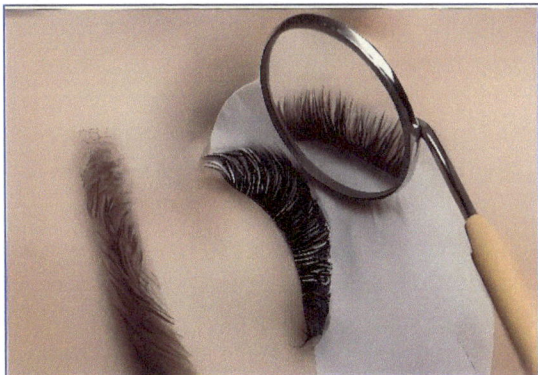

Then lift the lashes to be certain they have not stuck to the bottom lashes nor the pad covering the bottom lashes. Dental mirrors are great for checking your work.

Remember to have the client, move a few times during the process. About every- fifteen minutes or so.

Change their pillows or fluff the pillows up again. They can become very sore and stiff from laying there so still for such a long time.

For people with a full face the lash sizes will be longer from the outside and graduate down to 8 mm long lashes on the inner part of the eye near the nose. This type of shaping suits almost all face shapes.

However, for an aged face it is often best to make the longer lashes in the middle of each eye.

The best way to determine what suits the client and what is best for them is to hold a set of false lashes on one eye and ask what they think. Then a different shape, false lash on their eye.

The glue can feel brittle after a week or so. Therefore you need to be sure not to put the new lash near the skin and be certain you have very little glue on the lash. So, little you cannot actually see the glue. Believe me. It is so irritating that you will be constantly scratching the roots of your lashes. One time I felt as though I had tiny pieces of steel toughing my eyes. The therapist had put the glue too close to my eyelash roots and she used glue to make the lashes look thicker. I loved the look of my lashes but the irritation was too much to bear. No did she ask my permission to run glue the full length of the lashes to make them look thicker.

For this reason I had to have the extensions removed a week after they were done. I was not happy as it was Christmas time. I was on holidays and I had paid top dollar to look good for the festive season.

Never put more lashes than 30 on each eye. They will be too heavy.

After the glue has dried on both eyes show the client.

Should the client want more lashes you can then begin your second layer. However, if this is the clients 1st time at having eyelash

extensions then suggest she come back in a week time for another layer.

Below in this photo consider the black is the natural lash and the red is the added lash. In this photo all these positions are incorrect.

These positions (in red) are all wrong.

Care more so the client sings your praises.

Lets say the black lines are eyelashes and the red lines are the grafted lashes

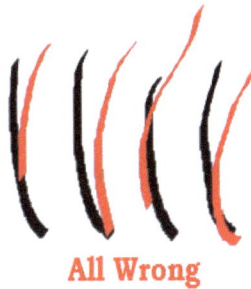

All Wrong

Below under the heading "Begin Eyelash Extensions" is your procedure sheet. Always check your tray set up and your procedure sheet before you begin.

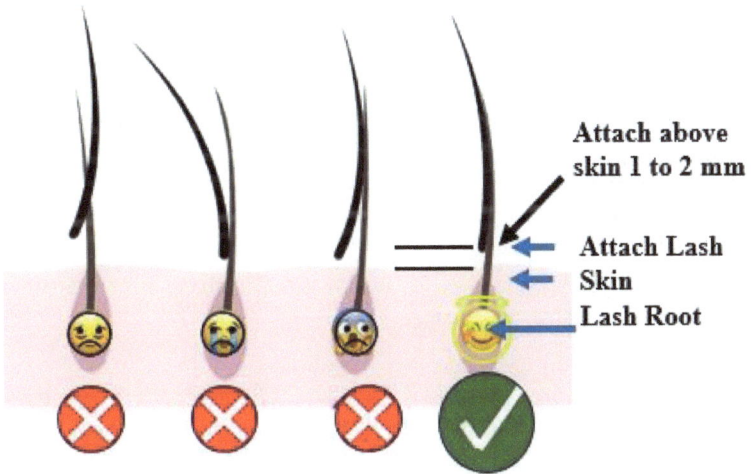

Attach above skin 1 to 2 mm

Attach Lash
Skin
Lash Root

This diagram -. Demonstrates a perfect joining point, a few millimetres from the natural lash base. Also, the glue must not noticeable at the join.

Every salon should have a procedures manual. In that manual under each heading you should have a procedure and tray set up for every service you offer in your salon. If you have staff they should study the manual and be quizzed from time to time on the procedures and tray set ups. You should never expect that they will get all the answers right. After all that is why you have the manual. The manual also helps the single operated salons to always get it right.

The most important fact is: knowing where the information is. When you quiz your staff you should observe who brings the manual to the meeting and who does not.

I would tell my staff we are going to have an open book quiz. I always ran the quiz before work.

How many times in your work day have you forgotten to put something important for the service on your tray?

You are setting up the room and you are called away to answer a clients question or to take a telephone call.

We are distracted many times when we are busy. Procedure manuals keep us professional.

The quiz time gives you the opportunity to observe those that know how to reference the notes they need in a heartbeat and those that barely have a clue. They are the ones that are not using the manual because they know it all. They are the staff member that all too often makes mistakes.

EYELASH PROTOCOL SHEET

This is your procedure sheet. Always check your tray set up and your procedure sheet before you begin. For new clients always do a patch test at least 24 hours beforehand.

Before you begin set up your work area.

Take a close up photo of the clients' eyes and add to her file.

Fill in the client form.

Check to see what size and thickness of lashes, you should use on the client.

Show her a few photographs of your work.

Hold a set of false lashes on one eye so she can judge the length and thickness.

Lay the client on a comfortable bed. In the beauty slant position.

Your stool must have wheels so you can move around the client with ease. Do not stand as you will not have the right type of control.

It is important that you do not use the clients face to control the balance of your hands. Use your torso. You can use your little finger as a pivot.

Never ever have the client sitting in a chair.

Be sure you have checked with the client as to how long she wants the lashes.

Place a few lashes on a smooth white makeup sponge.

Place the sponge on the bed near her head

Or if using the lashes that come in strips place them close to the clients head. You can place them on your wrist providing you have sterilized your hands and wrist well.

Now clean the eye area with cleaning fluid. The natural lashes must be soft and exceptionally free of oil.

Place a warm wet face pad on the clients closed eyes, followed by a cold wet cloth.

With the clients eyes open place a piece of glad wrap or masking tape over the bottom lashes.

Then brush the upper lashes to be sure the upper lashes are sitting above the glad-wrap and the lower lashes are sitting under the glad wrap.

It is important that you are able to comb the natural lashes without feeling any knots. If you are doing refills this is somewhat difficult. More care is required but still must be done.

Prime the lashes.

Put a tiny amount of glue onto a piece of glass or a Jade pad. Place the glass close to the client on the bed or their chest, on paper towel.

Care more so the client sings your praises.

Ask the client to close their eyes and keep them closed for the entire procedure.

Use your tweezers to push the lashes away from where you are going to apply the grafted lash.

One lash only must be between the tweezers. This lash must be in the Telogen stage of growth.

Pick up the thin end of the lash and dip the thicker end into some glue. Less is best.

When you have dipped the eyelash in glue, brush the excess glue off the lash extension. You do this by wiping the lash end on glass or eye pad.

Run the glue that is on the new lash up the length of the clients own eyelash. Do not get the glue on their lid shin.

Apply the lash to one of the client's lashes about **1 mm** up the lash. Not at the root but close to the root. This lash should have been chosen and separated from the other lashes before you grab the graft lash and before you dip the graft lash in the clue.

Never ever touch the skin with the glue.

Keep infilling each eye a few at a time on one eye then a few on the other eye. Never ever complete one eye first.

Repeat this process until you have 25-30 lashes on both eyes.

When you have completed the lashes use a hand blower to dry the lashes.

Do not use a hair dryer. The dryer below is also used for drying photos.

Now separate all the lashes with your tweezers.

Then lift the lashes to be certain they have not stuck to the bottom lashes or the pad covering the bottom lashes.

Remember to have the client, move a few times during the process. About, every fifteen minutes or so.

Change their pillows and fluff the pillows up again.

Never put more lashes than 30 on each eye. They will be too heavy.

After the glue has dried on both eyes Be sure to place a cold pack on her eyes for a few minutes..

Rinse her eyes with the saline mix.

Place mild eye drops in her eyes.

Check her eyes after asking her to blink several times.

Show the client her completed lashes.

Should the client want more lashes you can then begin your second layer. You must advise her that 25 to 30 lashes is best to allow her own lash cycle to perform the natural growth cycle and to allow for infills.

Care more so the client sings your praises.

More lashes causes growth cycle issuers. Such as the telogen lashes are the lashes you need to attach infill to. How many talogen stage lashes they have depends on how thick their natural lashes are.

THE MOST IMPORTANT STEPS

Charmlash, have a few tutorial videos you will find helpful.

https://charmlash.com/mistakes-to-avoid-during-lash-extension-removal/

FIRST STEP

The first most important step is the "Correct Position" I the author am assuming you have done a patch test on a new client.

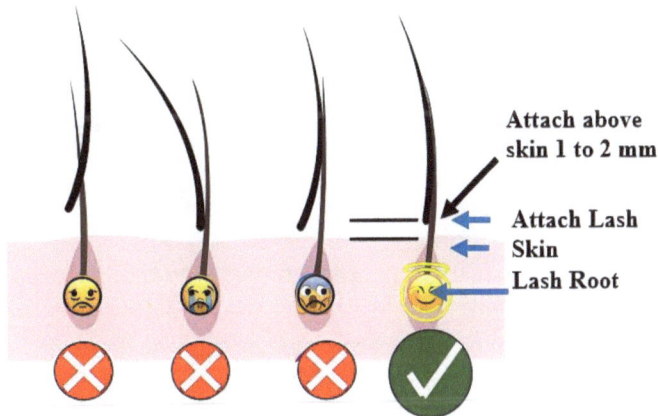

This position is correct. Place the lash extension onto the natural lash slightly above the root. Also be sure it contours against the natural lash. They should be attached to at least 85% of the natural lash.

You can dip the lash base into the glue then stroke the natural lash all the way up the lash with the glue that is on the extension. Then position the extension 1-2 mm up from the root. So that glue pooling does not occur always stroke the glue tip of the extension on the pad before applying the extension to the natural lash.

Remembering not to - ever put glue on the root of the natural lash nor on the skin of the eyelid. You must start 1 to 3 mm above the natural lash root.

There are many dangers when you do not get this position absolutely correct. Also, be very careful not to attach a graft lash to a new natural, baby lash. If you attach extensions to baby lashes there will be no new healthy lash cycle. Use good magnifying glasses so you can see clearly the different growth cycle of natural lashes. It is best to attach a graft to the Telogen stage lashes.

Photo of new lash with graft attached. **Do not attach a new graft to this lash** as it is in a Catagen lash (Transition) Phase:

The catagen phase is also known as the transition phase. During this phase, the lash stops growing and the hair follicle shrinks. If an eyelash falls out or is plucked out during this phase, it won't grow back right away because the follicle needs to complete the catagen phase before it can move on to the next one.

You can recognize this stage as these are the longest lashes on a client.

Care more so the client sings your praises.

This phase lasts between two and three weeks. Another - important reason - to buy an exceptional medical grade, pair of magnifying glasses.

It is important to know the difference between a catagen stage lash and an extension that is growing out. **Do not add a new extension to the one that is growing out.** As illustrated in the next photo.

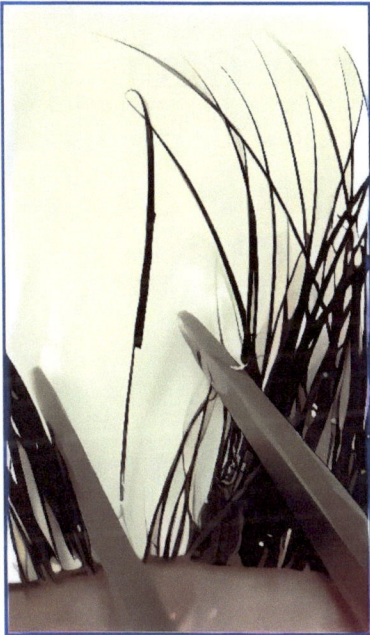

SECOND STEP

The Second Most Important Steps
Be sure the lash is sitting with the curve the same way as the natural lash curves. Sometimes when you pick the extension lash up with the tweezers you need to use your fingers to sit the lash in the tweezers the right way.

If you get this step right they will have great lashes that stay on for at least 2 months.

Providing you are attaching to a lash in Telogen stage. However, they will need to have infill's done during that time. The clients own natural eyelashes will fall out and hence the extension will go with it. Then a new lash will grow in the same place. The less glue you use the better.

THE AMOUNT OF GLUE

This is very bad.

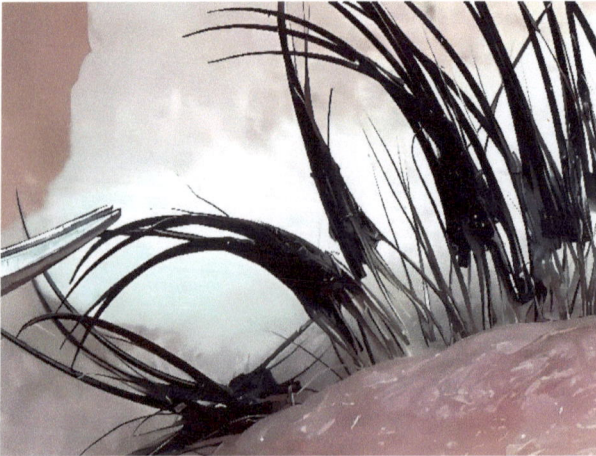

This is Fairly good

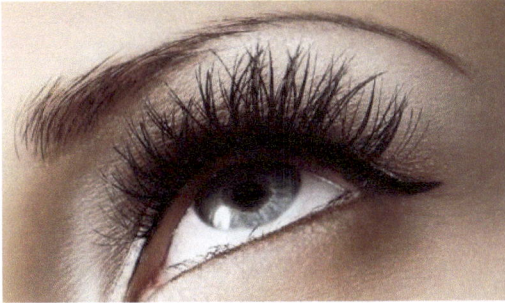

Now the lashes need brushing to form a better shape and may need to be combed with a warm wand. Be careful wands tend to curl the lashes and curly lashes are hard to work on.
Plus wands melt glue.

Note:
The therapist in the above photo has tattooed the eyeliner close to the lashes on the outer side of the eye. Then she tattooed the inner part of the eye, **inside** the eye. That is illegal in Australia and as our standards are recognized internationally I would think it is illegal everywhere.

This is better

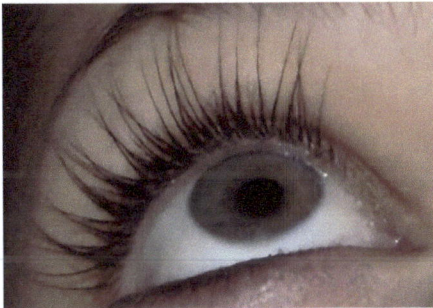

There are only a few lashes that have a tiny bit too much glue. The above photo "after" photo is a job well done. Note: the new anagen (baby eyelashes) have not had extensions attached to. The glue is a few millimetres away from the root of the natural lash.

Below in the next photo the student has placed too much glue on these extensions. If you look closely she has also put glue onto the skin and the Distichiasis lashes.

With every lash you apply check that there is no pooling of glue. Use toothpicks if you have applied to much glue to remove the excess while you hold the neighbouring lashes away with the tweezers.

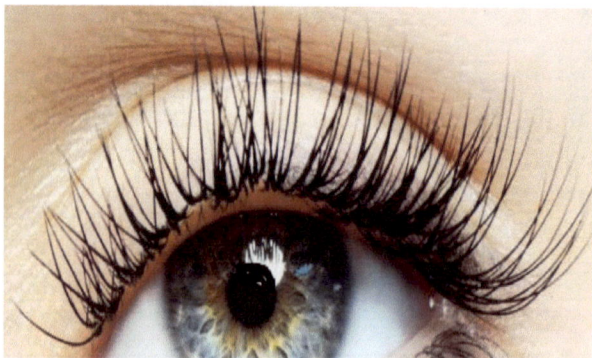

On this client, the student put the glue too close to the root. It is very messy. On further observations - it appears there has been grafted lashes added to some of the new baby lashes.

This is dangerous as it prevents the growth pattern forming correctly. It is imperative not to attach grafted lashes to the new baby lashes.

Care more so the client sings your praises.

This client has **distichiasis** and it appears extensions have been added to the lashes under the root line to the distichiasis lashes. Pus the glue is too thick.

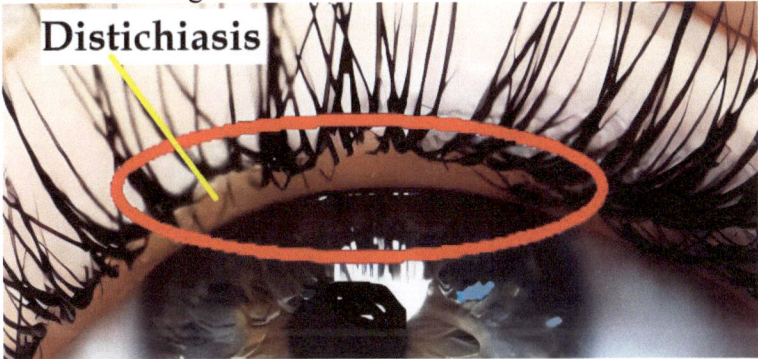

Separating the lashes. You need to practice - how to get this step right. This helps you to prevent glue attaching to nearby lashes.

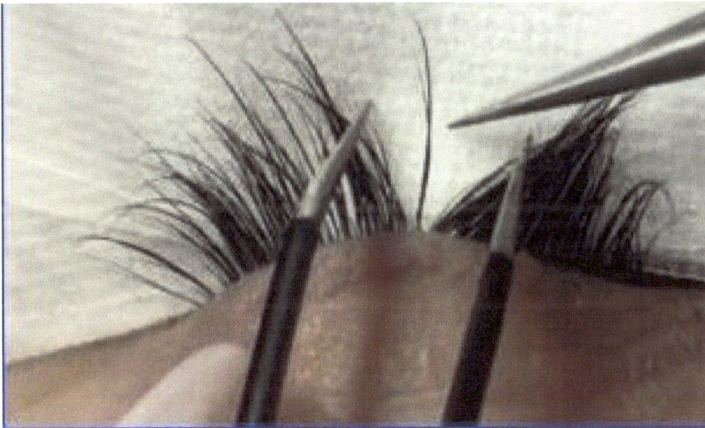

Next two photos - dip in glue
Then wipe glue off extension.

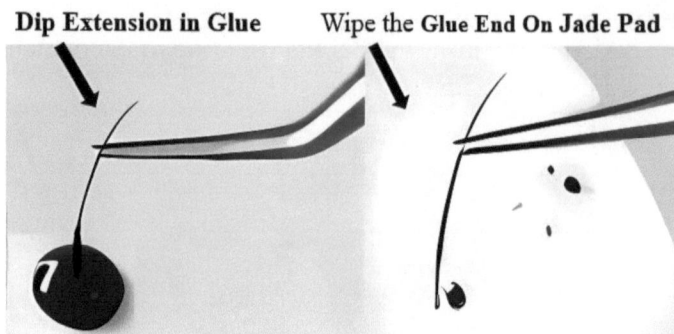

Watch lash extensions on YouTube. You will soon get to know which videos are excellent and the ones that are a disgrace to our trade.

THIRD STEP

The Third Important Step is:-
"The Amount of Glue." Which is by far the very most important step. Too much glue causes problems. Get this wrong and the glue will irritate the eye. It could even cause damage to the delicate skin and the eyeball. After a day or two the glue sets so hard it is like fine strips of Steele.

You place a small drop of glue onto a small glass plate.

Pick up the lash in the middle of the lash or the middle of the bunch of lashes. This will depend on whether you are applying single lashes or applying bunches of lashes.

When you dip the thick end of the lash extension into the glue, be certain to wipe it on the jade pad as it needs to be just a tiny amount of glue on the base of the lash.

Learn More to Earn More

With eyelash grafting be sure that only one of the clients natural lashes is between the tweezers.

With a stroking motion attach the lash extension 2 to 3 mm from the natural lash root.

Be sure the lash sits along the natural lash.

When you attach a couple of lashes use a tooth pick to roll off the excess glue from the underside of the lashes. The toothpick should only be used once and then a new one used on the next few lashes. I actually do this with every bunch I place on the lashes.

Look under the lashes often. .
It is important they are not sticking to the pad

Both the bunch and the natural lash should be in a "C" or "J" shape running up towards the eyebrow.

All the same rules apply for bunches of lash as for grafted lashes. Do not apply too close to the skin. Do not apply to baby lashes.

Note: Some peoples natural lashes have a few lashes that are sun damaged and curl downwards. In this case you will need to curly their lashes with a warm curling wand before you begin. However, this can also cause more difficulty when aligning the lashes.

You will need a supply of different shapes and of a variety of thicknesses.

Watch This video on YouTube.
https://www.youtube.com/watch?v=AfWEpUCV_cA

The therapist in this video, does a lovely job. She does not dry the lashes with the blower but I feel she has done a perfect job in every other way.

EYELASH GLUE

Cautions:

- Buy glue for professional use only
- Check ingredients list methodically.
- Eyes must remain closed during entire procedure
- Keep glue in cool and dry place
- Avoid direct sunlight
- Shake well before using
- Do not store in the refrigerator.
- Keep out of reach of children
- Avoid contact with skin
- In case of contact with eyes, flush with saline solution for 10 minutes and consult a physician immediately.

Never ever keep any glue in the refrigerator.

 I have not checked the ingredients of all glue types. I know that Blinks "Advanced Glue" has Cyano Acrylate in it. Therefore, I would not use it - if I was still working in the industry. They have lots of other glues, so check out their ingredients.

Learn More to Earn More

As you would know I am now retired therefore, I have not ordered glue for about six years. In 2007 my glue cost me about $125 and is no longer on the market.

Eyelash glue has come down in price and has improved considerably. It has been my experience in my life that the more people in your industry you associate with the more you feed off each others knowledge. Ask other therapist what they are using and what kind of results they are having with that product. But still check the ingredients list.

Have your eyebrows waxed regularly at other salons. This way you get to meet other beauty therapist and build a rapport or friendship and talk about products. If your supplier is not a therapist they will only be giving you the information they have been feed - by the manufacturer.

First be sure to choose the right glue. Latex rubber based glue is what most suppliers offer. You need to find glue with no Formaldehyde or Cyano Acrylate. I know that Blinks Advanced glue has Cyano Acrylate in it. Be sure to ask questions about their other types of glue.

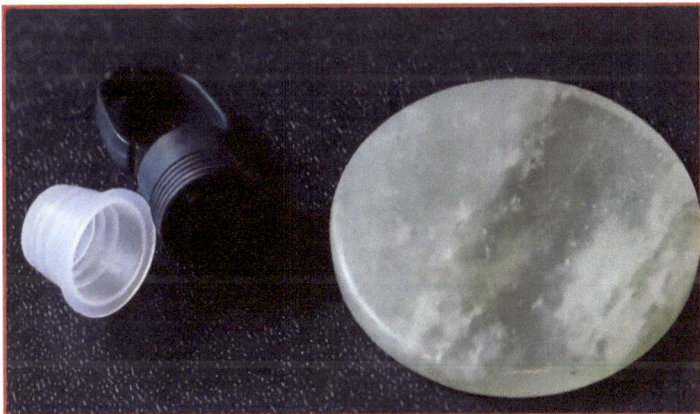

Ring, Ring Cup and Jade Stone Pad. The glue can be placed in a ring or on a stone pad or a small piece of glass.

Some salon eyelash glue contains dangerous chemicals such as Formaldehyde. Other salon suppliers have eyelashes glue or adhesives that contain Cyano Acrylate.

Abstract
From http://www.ncbi.nlm.nih.gov/pubmed/17388821

Cyanoacrylate (CA) and its homologues have a variety of medical and commercial applications as biological adhesives and sealants. Homologues of CA are being widely promoted in surgery as a tissue adhesive to replace traditional suturing techniques. Potential benefits of using CA adhesives include better cosmetic results, more rapid wound closure, and perhaps most significantly, the potential for significant reductions in percutaneous injuries from suture needles, which would in turn also reduce the risk of transmission of infectious diseases.

Nevertheless, certain concerns have been raised regarding the potential toxicity of CA within patients, as well as among health professionals who are occupationally exposed when using CA compounds.

Reported toxicity of CA in the workplace may result in dermatological, allergic and respiratory conditions. To help reduce the occupational burden, therefore, medical staff using CA adhesives should avoid direct contact with the compound and use appropriate personal protective measures at all times. Maintaining higher levels of humidity, optimizing room ventilation and using special air conditioning filters in surgical suites and operating theatres may also be useful in minimizing the exposure to volatile CA adhesives.

The above **Abstract** should give you an idea of the type of research you should do about what you are placing on your client and the effects these product have on you and other salon members.

The semi permanent eyelash glue can be hard to remove and eventually clients will pull out their own eyelashes. Try to find special eyelash adhesive that has no Formaldehyde or Cyano Acrylate.

However, the bond is not as long lasting. I recommend using the stronger glue but if the eyelash glue becomes too brittle then it must be remove with olive oil. If you have attached the extension at least 3mm from the eyelash root the hardened glue is often **not** a major problem. Closer to the skin and it will be like Steel rubbing our eyes.

If it is causing eye irritation - rub each lash with fingers to create a friction on the lash and ease off. Then clean the lashes with a warm soap and water mix. Baby shampoo is known not to cause eyes to burn and therefore is a good eyelash cleanser when used on a cotton tip and rolled gently on the roots. Hold a timber tongue depressor under the lashes.

Leave lashes off for a few weeks then start again. I have been having my lashes done for many years and yes sometimes my own lashes come out but I still have plenty not that I ever had great lashes.

Most of the lashes do grow back if the therapist stays away from the eyelash root with the glue and pays particular attention to which lash she attaches the extension to. *See heading "Lash Growth Cycle".*

See below for more information on eyelash removal.

I repeat. ***Do not allow the glue to touch the eyelash skin or the eyelash root.***

I have found that the most expensive glues are not what they say they are. I have paid one hundred and twenty five dollars for extension glue and it was not as good as the glue I paid seventy five dollars for. They have come down in price over the years. They now sell glue for around forty dollars. Be sure to check the ingredients list. Then Google the ingredient names on the list.

If the ingredients are safe it does not matter what the price is.

The Golden Rule with Glue

1. **Less is best.**
2. **Never place the glue on the natural lash root.**
3. Never get the glue on the eyelid skin.

BEAUTY SLANT POSITION

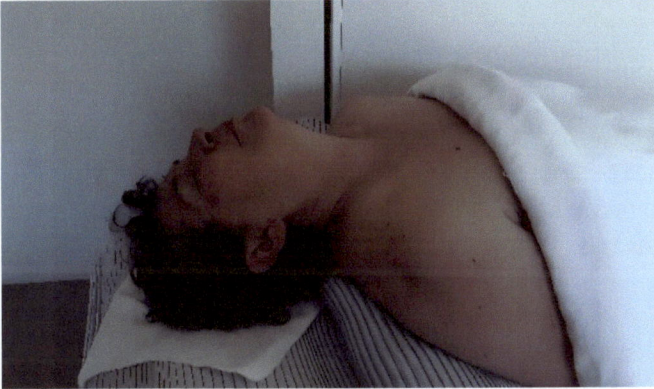

We talk about the beauty slant position throughout all my Beauty School Books. The clients head must be tilted back so the eyes are in line with their shoulders.

Place an extra pillow under her shoulders and ask if he/she is comfortable.

Your stool should have wheels so you can move easily around the client.

The bed should be lowered so the clients eyes are at your elbow height when you are sitting. This gives you better control.

Natural Eye Cleansing Solution:

Clean Eye Using Natural Eye Cleansers

The eyes are very important parts of our body. Any problem that we have in our eyes will make daily living very difficult. There are many known natural eye cleansing solution today, and because they are natural, it readily means that they are safe.

You will need to clean the clients eyes after the eyelash extensions and they may need to flash their eyes the next day.

Saline Recipe

A solution of distilled water or boiled water and table salt is also effective. Just mix one cup of water with half a teaspoon of salt. If you are using boiled water, be sure to let it cool before placing in storage containers.

Store in food safe plastic squirt style bottles. Beauty suppliers call them "Neutralizer bottles." But you need to ask if they are food safe plastic. You can keep for 2 days.

Green Tea Eye Rinse

Another natural eye cleansing solution is the mixture of one-part distilled water and two parts green tea. This green tea eye wash solution is popular for making the eye feel refreshed, and it relieves itchiness and irritation. Others also apply teabags immediately on closed eyes to reduce swelling and lighten dark circles.

Chamomile Is Healing.

Chamomile is a daisy-like plant that is widely known for its many therapeutic uses and a natural eye cleanser. It is effective for burning, itching, and dry red eyes. Follow these steps to make an eye cleanser:
Pour boiled water into the chamomile tea bag in a cup.
Let it stand for two to five minutes.
Remove the tea bag and let the tea cool.
It is best when at the same as your body temperature or make sure that the eyes can tolerate it.
Put a towel under a kidney bowl on the clients face at the corner of their eye. Their head should be laying towards the beauty bed. Squirt a little in the eye then a little more. Pat with soft cotton wool pad.

Beauty suppliers also have single use eye cleaners.

TIPS TO CLEANSE EYE

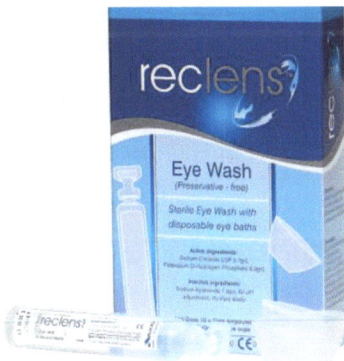

Furthermore, here are tips to clean eyes naturally using the above solutions:

Do not clean both eyes at the same time. Instead, close one eye (for instance the left eye) and pour the solution carefully from the corner of the right eye near the nose. Do the same thing for the other eye.

Never use any of the solutions for 6 hours from the time they have been made. They might be contaminated with microorganisms that can cause eye infections.

Always use distilled or boiled water. Tap water has various elements that can further complicate the eye problem.

Tips to clean the eyes naturally include the use of clean materials and proper hygiene.

REMOVING EYELASH EXTENSIONS

First rule encourage the client to remove them slowly herself over several weeks with olive oil and brushing. There are many dangers when removing extensions. All removal products have acetone in them.

How to remove the extensions will depend greatly on how much glue was applied and what type of glue was used.

To remove eyelash extensions is somewhat dangerous. You must protect the clients delicate skin around the eyes and their eyes. The removers can be very harsh.

If you have been the technician to apply the lashes as per the instructions in this manual then the job should be easy.

First clean the clients face and eye area.

Then use a gentle toner to complete the cleaning process.

Cover the eye lid and the bottom lashes with tape and cotton pads.

Place a warm wet face cloth on the eyes for a few minutes.

Soak a cotton ball with olive oil. Wipe it on the lashes, taking care not to get any in their eye. Continue gently wiping the lashes with oil until the extensions begin to fall off.

You can remove them by gently rubbing with olive oil mixed with ground sea salt. Mix 2 tablespoons olive oil with quarter teaspoon of ground salt. Bush onto eyelashes then use your fingers to run the lashes without rubbing the eye shin.

You may need to use a disposable mascara wand to assist with the breaking of the glue bond. I use two brushes one each side of the lashes and use a friction movement with the lashes between the brushes.

If the glue is thick and hard to remove you will need to use eyelash extension glue remover. However, this is not advisable as it stings and damages the delicate skin on the eye lids.

Remove all the olive oil with a warm face cloth and then use a drop of toner on a cotton bud and clean the lashes.

I recommend having the client wash her face over your basin with a liquid cleanser and warm water to complete the cleaning process.

If you intend to clean her face and charge her be sure to rinse her face extremely well.

Eyelash Grafting and Party Lashes

Dry her face.

Have her get comfortable again on the bed.

Place a drop of olive oil on a cotton tip and smooth over the delicate eye skin close to but not on the lashes. Wait a few minutes and tap around the delicate eye area to bring more blood and oxygen to the skin surface. Then apply a warm wet face cloth. Next apply a cold pack.

Reapply cotton pads to beneath her bottom lashes and to her eyelid.

Place a small amount of glue remover to a disposable mascara wand. Remember I have said before, glue remover is very hash and I try never ever to use it.

Try very hard not to get the glue remover on the skin. This is a complete work of art so put on your magnifying goggles.

With your pointy finger and your thumb, press down on the cotton pad so it will not move.

With the wand in the other hand firmly and slowly brush down on the top lashes.

Then use the eyelash comb to comb the lashes. It will be a slow and tedious job. For this reason be sure to explain the cost to your client.

I recommend you write an eyelash removing leaflet and give to clients with a small kit.

The kit would contain:-

Learn More to Earn More

1. Four cotton pads
2. Three disposable wands
3. Two eye pads
4. Saline

They should attempt to remove the eyelashes them self at home with warm olive oil on a wand. If they are patient this is the best method.

They should put the olive oil in an oil burner or put oil on a one tablespoon and hold a match under the spoon to warm it. They can dip the wand in the oil.
Test the heat on your wrist before applying to the lashes.

Note: some people say to heat the lashes as this softens the glue. Oh yes it will if you keep it going until the eyes almost burn.

Glue sets like a rock after a day or so this is why less is best. You will never ever loosen the glue with heat. A warm cloth is to sooth the eyes not loosen or soften the glue. It will soften it the tiniest bit but not enough to remove the glue. Heat will only work if the lashes were glued on in the last hour or so. Extensions and false eyelash glue are two different molecular structures.

Structure and Shape Effects of Molecular Glue on Supramolecular Tubulin Assemblies

Is not a subject we even touch on in beauty training, is it now? If they did add it to beauty training they would have to add, at the very least another 150 hours to the course to even touch the surface of the types of bonds used in glue.

Am I equipped to touch on this subject? Hell no. However, I have used enough types of glue to know I hate them being used on our eyelashes. Can I recommend a great eyelash glue? No. After five decades of trying glues I am still not satisfied that a glue manufacturing company has even tried to produce a safe glue for us.

The only help I can give you is to warn you not to get it on the skin and to keep the glue 1-3 mm away from the lash root when applying lashes. Don't try to repair other peoples mistakes get the client to remove them herself.

When I listen to the sales blubs at Beauty Expo I am greatly amused. I also think to myself. I have been there done that. I too have had blind, uneducated faith in what my suppliers tell me. The older we get the more we realize how little we know.

I like the video that this therapist has produced so watch her removing lashes.

http://www.wikihow.com/Remove-Eyelash-Extensions

 I checked this video on the 30th July 2015 and it is still working. Rechecked February 2019 and still working.

My only constructive criticism is she did not apply a pad to the upper lid nor a protective layer of oil. No strips of tape to keep the eyes firm.

These strips pull the eye skin taut and away from the lashes. They should be applied no matter how firm the clients skin is.

I dislike the use of petroleum jelly and baby oil which is a mineral oil. However, in this case for eyelash removal they are a great product to protect the delicate eye area while removing lashes. Be very sparing and only give the eyes a tiny coat of one of these.

This is a well trained therapist. After searching for three hours to find a video I could recommend to you, this therapist was the best I found. July 2010.

TEST 1 EYELASH EXTENSIONS

Eyelash Certificate Students only to do this test. However, it will assist everyone wanting to apply lash extensions. The only difference is: - you will not have a teacher to debate the videos with.

Look up a few YouTube sites on eyelash extensions and email us the addresses to look at. Most movies go for 1-3 minutes. Your teacher will also look at the sites you have looked at and give you feed back on what they did right and wrong on the video you watched.

Take at least seven points from the ABOVE information and make an eye care sheet to give your clients. Send a copy to your teacher.

I have supplied one for you to view and the address of one video.

Understand this before you read my comments. When making videos the therapist is nervous. They also have to consider where the camera is so they are working in unnatural conditions. Under these circumstances they are doing a great job.

WATCH MOVIE CLIP ON GRAFTING

http://www.europeanbeautyconcept.com/

Copy and paste this site address into your web browser.
Click on Eyelashes
Click on educational movie.

This therapist opened three jars of lashes. Only open one at a time and put the lid back on straight away.
Place the lashes on a sponge.

Have a different sponge colour for each size lash. Then open the next jar with the next size lash, then the third jar with the next size lashes.

Place the pads with the lashes on, in sized order. Or buy them in strips but this is more expensive and sometimes they are very hard to get off the strip.

HOW TO SUBMIT YOUR EXAMS

Only do this test if you are doing a full course with Beauty School Books.

Note: Here at Beauty School Books we are not an accredited beauty school and we only cater for students that are unable to attend a beauty school.

Email answers to or mailto:beautyschoolbooks@gmail.com

Learn More to Earn More

If you are training yourself you can request some video conference time with me for a small fee. Use Skype as the carrier.

If you have already been trained and you are reading this book to improve your skills you are to be congratulated.

If you are training at a beauty school you should feel very proud. There is no better way to train than to attend a quality school.

In the subject line put the course name and the test name.

In the body put your student header sheet with your personal details.

Then attach the test answers.

Your header sheet must contain;-

The test and course name
Your name
Date of Birth
Address
Telephone
Email address.

FORMS FOR CLIENT

The first thing you need to understand is this is a training manual I cannot possible set it all out for you in the manual. Some people may need this manual delivered as an eBook. All eBook readers are different sizes so I am limited to formatting requirements. However, I am happy to email forms to you. There is a small fee.

Please adjust to suit client having Eye Enhancement treatment. Then forward to your teacher for feedback.

Sample client treatment plan eye enhancement should contain:-

Name:
Address:
 Tel. Work:
Tel. Home:
Occupation:
D.O.B.:
Medical conditions:
Lifestyle factors:

Here you need to know about their sporting activities. If they swim a lot, ask them to keep their head above water for a few days and explain they may need more infills than another client.

General health: Excellent, good, poor
Medication
Known allergies:
Are you allergic to latex?
Ask all the illness questions.
Do you have AIDS,
 Hepatitis,
 Heart Condition,
 Do you faint?
Have Diabetes,
Eyes water a lot,
Conjunctivitis,

Care more so the client sings your praises.

Epileptic
Have you had Chemotherapy or radiation therapy in the last 12 months?
Have you taken any drugs today, when did you last have a drink of alcohol, yes/no
have many glasses,___ of what,_____
Skin type:
Skin condition:
 Skin Type: Combination,
 Dry,
Oily,
 Dark,
 Fair,
Olive,
Youthful,
 Mature,
Dehydrated
Notes:
Have you had lash done before?
When did you have a patch test done?___
If not we will need to perform a patch test prior to the applications. Appointment time for patch test is:
Previous treatments:
Contra-indications:
Comments / request
Treatment,
Therapist
 Date
Price
30 lashes /25 lashes
Second layer yes /no

Set the form up like this below picture.
 The more professionally your forms are set out the easier it will be for you to fill them in. The client expects to be asked questions.

When you also ask appropriate questions they feel they are in the hands of a professional.

Make the form very quick and easy to fill in with lots of yes and no answers. That way it will be quick to fill in. If you have to write down all their answers it could take an hour.

Name:			
Address:		Tel Work:	Tel Home:
Occupation:		D.O.B:	
Medical conditions:		Lifestyle factors:	
		Here you need to know about their sporting activities. If they swim a lot ask them to keep their head above water for a few days and explain they may need more infills than another client.	
General health: ☐ excellent ☐ good ☐ poor	Medication:	Known allergies:	
Skin type:	Skin condition:	Notes:	
☐ normal	☐ blemished	☐ coupe rose	
☐ oily	☐ dehydrated	☐ prematurely aged	
☐ dry	☐ sensitive	☐ other	
☐ combination	☐ mature	☐ Eye water a lot	
Previous treatments:			
Body condition:		Postural conditions:	
Contra-indications:			
Comments / requests:			
TREATMENT	THERAPIST	DATE	PRICE
30 lashes /25 lashes			

You can set this type of form pictured here in the program called Excel. Add your disclaimer at the bottom of the Clients form.

Care more so the client sings your praises.

Learn More to Earn More

Test Two,

PRACTICE EYELASH EXTENSION.

Watch four YouTube videos.
 Paste their address into a word document and write your comments on what you feel they did right and what you feel they did wrong.

Send to your teacher for her to watch and see if she agrees with your comments. If you do not have a personal trainer for this subject then at least you will have made the effort to improve your skills.
Then watch those movies again in a month time after you have studied and practiced some more.

PRACTICE ON FALSE EYELASHES.

For practice start with lashes similar to 1 or 2 in the top row of this picture.

Practice on a set of false eyelashes. When you first start it is easier to glue the false lashes to an orange or the dolls forehead. Also use two pins at each end to keep the false lashes laying firm on the orange or doll.

After you feel confident - with the use of your tools and separating the lashes. Glue a set of false lashes on a dolls eye and perform the extensions.

1. Set up everything you need onto a tray.
2. The more you practice before doing them on humans the better.
3. Check your work the next day comb the lashes to see if they all stay on
4. Check that the glue is almost invisible to see.
5. Check the glue is at least 2-3 mm away from the band on the false lashes.

6. Check that you have not glued the new extension to more than one lash on the false lashes.

It is important to realize that you are going to be using tools and products in a way you have not experienced before. While practicing on false lashes you will be tempted to move them to a convenient position. In a real situation you will not be able to move the clients head to suit your hand movements.

After you become familiar with your tools then practice on a dolls head.
Put the dolls head on a massage bed. Attach false lashes.
Now practice adding single extensions to the false lashes, as though you are working on a client.

EYE ANATOMY

To become an eyelash grafting / extension therapist you must hold either a certificate in beauty therapy or a diploma.

EYE SKIN CARE & ANATOMY

Our skin is the largest organ of our body, not all parts of our skin is created with same character. The skin on the scalp has embedded hair follicles; the skin of the nose and cheeks tends to have active glands.

The skin around your eyes is very sensitive and delicate, which needs good care no matter what your age group is. Weather its summer or winter or any other season, follow some simple steps and guidelines as explained below, to have healthier skin around your eyes!

The skin has sweat glands and hairs. As the junction between skin and conjunctiva is approached, the hairs change their character to become eyelashes. Just like hair, the growth of your eyelashes occurs in cycles, which include a growing and a resting phase. At the end of the resting phase, the hair will fall out, meaning that new hair will soon come out. To give you an average estimate of how fast eyelashes grow back, it's anywhere from 1 to 6 weeks. Seldom is each lash on the same cycle, thank heavens. Therefore, most people do not notice when the eyelash skin is in the resting cycle. Just like farm land, a smart farmer knows when to rest his paddock and we should rest our eyes from lash extensions.

It is vitally important that the front surface of the eyeball, the cornea, remain moist. This is achieved by the eyelids, which during waking hours sweep the secretions of the lacrimal apparatus and other glands over the surface at regular intervals and which during sleep cover the eyes and prevent evaporation.

The lids have the additional function of preventing injuries from foreign bodies, through the operation of the blink reflex. The lids are essentially folds of tissue covering the front of the orbit and, when the eye is open, leaving an almond-shaped aperture. The points of the almond are called canthi;

Now even though the eyes should be moist they should not be weeping in anyway.

The 1st thing an Eyelash technician should do is shine a torch into the client's eyes. If the clients eyes weep or

water up - do not do the grafting on this client. They may have a weak eye condition. Most eyes will water from the glue fumes and this can be avoided by keeping their eyes closed during the procedure and for 5 to 10 minutes after the procedure.

Growth is the progressive development of a living being or part of an organism from its earliest stage to maturity. Development involves the series of changes by which the individual embryo becomes a mature organism.

THE BASIC PROCESSES OF CELL GROWTH ARE:

CELL DIVISION (MULTIPLICATION)

Cell division occurs throughout a human's life. In any animal, cells are constantly divided to form more cells, either to add new tissue to the existing organism or to replace damaged tissue. This kind of cell division is called mitosis.

CELL DIFFERENTIATION

Cell differentiation is the process by which a general cell type changes to form a cell type with a specialised function.

Although the process for the way that cells achieve this is unknown, it is generally believed that it involves switching mechanisms in the nucleus of the cell. Some pieces of the information contained in the DNA within the nucleus are turned off while others are turned on. Thus, although cell with a nucleus has the same chromosomes and DNA, different cells use different parts of that information just as different students will use different sections of a library.

Care more so the client sings your praises.

THE GROWTH OF THE EPIDERMIS

The diagram below shows the different stages in the growth of the epidermis.

1. The layer of stem cells in the germinative layer of the epidermis

2. Cells produced in the germinative layer are pushed towards the surface, become flattened and die.

    The remains of the cells lose their identity and become converted into layers of keratin. Eventually,

3. these flakes of keratin are lost from the surface of the skin.

4. For better looking skin it is important for us to give these dead cells a helping hand to dissipate. Which is done - by exfoliating our skin, during the cleansing process.

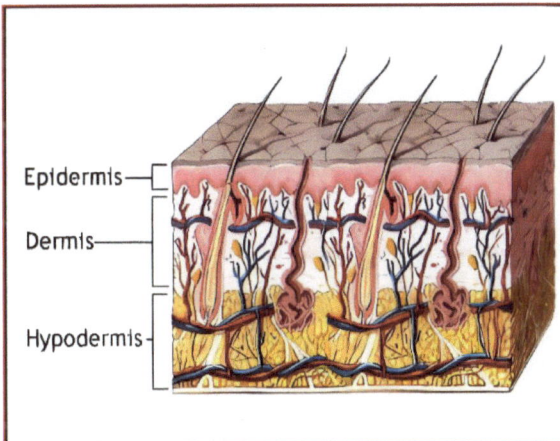

5. Dead cells need to be removed every week from our skin to slow down the aging process. Under a microscope they like fish scales in the Stratum Corneum layer.

The Anatomy of the Skin Around the Eyes

Students you do not want to make money at the expense of harm - to your client's eyes. Study the skin and lashes. We have supplied you with a brief explanation but you as a caring person will study the eyes in detail.

The glue you use to graft the lashes can cause eyes to burn. Make sure the client keeps their eyes closed for 10-15 minutes after the procedure so the glue is completely dry before they open their eyes.

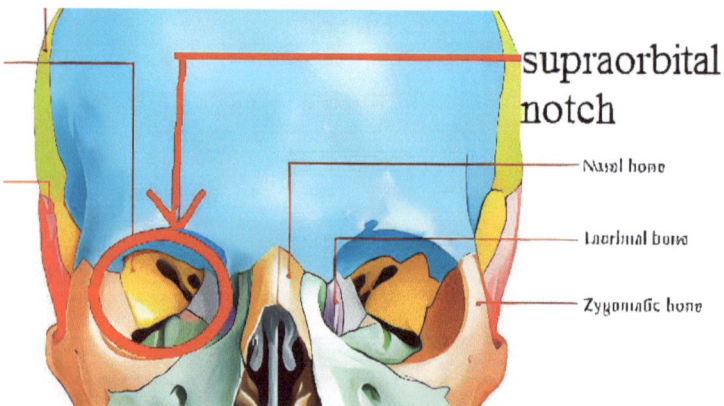

supraorbital notch

Nasal bone

Lacrimal bone

Zygomatic bone

Orbicularis Oculi muscles are circular sphincters which surround the eyes and close the eyelids. They relax when sleeping and can be used independently as when winking. The Pink area is the Levator Palpebrae Superioris muscles sit on the eyelids, open the eyelids and work as an antagonist to the Orbicularis Oculi the green area.

The Corrugator Supercilii muscles are located in the orbital arch and draw the eyebrows inwards and downwards causing the vertical lines on the forehead when frowning. Encourage your clients to gently massage this area daily.

The anatomy of the skin around the eyes, also referred to as the adnexa is unique to the face and body. In order to properly care for the skin around the eyes, it is important to understand not only the anatomy of this area, but also the process of skin cell renewal.

Eyelid skin is composed of several layers. The deepest, the subcutaneous layer contains a thin layer of fascia which lies on top of the orbicularis muscle, a muscle that allows the eyelid to move.

Next, the dermis, which forms the support layer of the skin, is made up of threadlike proteins including bundles of elastin and collagen, fibroblasts, nerves and vessels.

 The top layer, the epidermis, is made up of basal cells, melanocytes, Langerhans cells, keratinocytes and on top, the dead cell layer (also known as the stratum corneum) made up of corneocytes. The epidermal layer gives the skin its appearance, colour, suppleness, texture, and health.

Basal cells reproduce new cells every few days. As these cells migrate upward, they become drier and flatter. Once they reach the surface of the skin, they are no longer alive, and are referred to as corneocytes. This process of migration from basal cell to corneocytes is what gives the epidermis the ability to regenerate itself. This skin renewal process is known as desquamation.

Desquamation is an ongoing process that takes about two weeks in a young person, and significantly longer – about 37 days for individuals over 50. The build up of corneocytes gives skin a callous or dry, aged and thickened look. The skin feels and looks rough and its ability to retain water becomes impaired.

There are also clients that have very dry skin around the eyelash area. These clients may have mites in their lashes. Mites cannot be seen by the naked eye. I have submitted two photos for you to have a look at mites in lashes. These photos were taken under a microscope. The only way of knowing if the client has mites is a letter from an eye specialist. If the client eyes look dry or reddish, explain they have a dry eye condition.

They would not be able to have extensions without a clearance letter from an eye specialist. You are not an eye specialist so do not tell them what you think they have.

I have given you this information as a safety tool. You do not want to spread this disease to other clients. This is why the Australia Standards state that a trained Beauty Therapist with skin science knowledge perform the art of eyelash extensions.

EYE DISEASES

ALOPECIA:

Alopecia is the technical term for hair loss. There are many types of hair loss that can affect the eyelashes, but we will focus on the following two disorders:

Traction alopecia is a form of alopecia, or gradual hair loss, caused primarily by a pulling force being applied to the hair. When the hair is removed from the follicle prematurely, it causes the follicle to shrink. When this is done repeatedly, it could lead to permanent lash loss. In the case of lash extensions, you can be at fault for causing traction alopecia. Here's how you can do your part to make sure your client's lashes stay healthy and strong.

1. Applying lashes that are too heavy for the natural lash repeatedly can cause the natural lashes to prematurely shed. Keep in mind, a healthy lash can hold up to 30 grams of weight while a fine or fragile lash can only support approximately 15 grams of weight.
2. Applying more than one lash or one fan/bunch to one natural eyelash can cause pulling on an anagen lash that is not ready to shed. Remember that each one of our lashes is in its own individual growth cycle.

BLEPHARITIS

Is the chronic inflammation of the eyelids. It can be due to infection (staphylococcus, herpes, fungus, and others), seborrhoea, trauma (plucking, rubbing, bad applied extensions), or allergy (specially to cosmetics).

EYELASH MITES

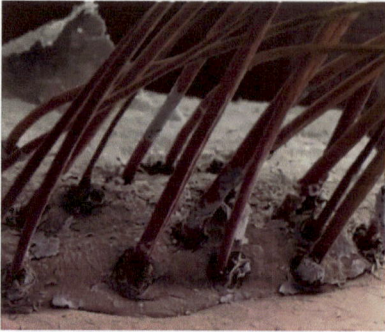

Lash mites on hair follicles − Courtesy of science photo library

Above Photo is of dry skin and lash mites on the hair / lash follicles. Blow are mites in the lash and root area. Both these photos have been taken under a microscope. You will not see the mites unless you have good magnifying glasses.

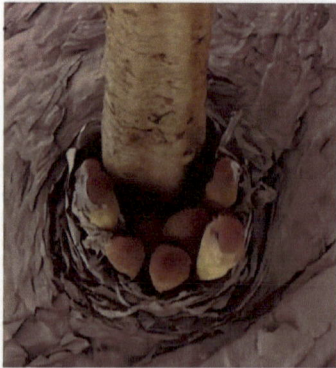

Eyelash mites infestation on eyelash follicle

Demodex mites are readily visualized under the microscope using the 4× objective lens; however, the 10× lens is recommended to enhance ease of detection of both mites and eggs.

.

CRAB LICE

These are parasitic insects which infest pubic zones and other areas, including eyelashes. They use to feed with human blood, and the treatment with Permethrin and Pyrethrins is hard, and should be completed with fine-teeth combs and washings.

DEMODEX FOLLICULORUM

These are parasites, face mites, who lives in the eyelashes follicles. They eat sebaceous secretions and dead cells, and they reproduce inside the follicle. With a length of 0.1 to 0.4 mm., they can infest the eyelids.

DISTICHIASIS

Photo credit -
https://emedicine.medscape.com/article/1212908-overview

Two types of distichiasis can be identified, acquired and congenital. In the acquired form, most cases involve the lower lids. Lashes can be fully formed or very fine, pigmented or non-pigmented, properly oriented or misdirected. The congenital form is dominantly inherited with complete penetrance. It can be isolated or associated with ptosis, strabismus, congenital heart defect, or mandibulofacial dysostosis. This defect may be related to the epithelial germ cells failure to differentiate completely to meibomian glands, instead they become pilosebaceous units.

Distichiasis can affect the lower and upper lids (see following image). Contact between abnormal lashes and the cornea can result in severe eye irritation or ulcers.

Eyelash Grafting and Party Lashes

ENTROPION

Entropion is a malposition resulting in inversion of the eyelid margin. The morbidity of the condition is a result of ocular surface irritation and damage.

Successful management of this condition depends on appropriate classification and a procedural choice that adequately addresses the underlying abnormality.

Naturally it is advisable to encourage clients with these eye disorders and other eye diseases not to have eyelash extensions.

It is assumed you have studied eye disorders during you Beauty Diploma study. For those of you without a diploma it is best to research all eye conditions and to understand causes and effects.

MADAROSIS

Also known as milphosis, is the abnormal loss of eyelashes (Ciliary Madarosis). It could be caused by inflammation (blepharitis), alopecia, tumours, endocrine disorders, congenital disorders, drugs and toxins, or wrong applied make up or extensions.

PATHOPHYSIOLOGY

is the study of the changes of normal mechanical, physical, and biochemical functions, either caused by a disease or resulting from an abnormal syndrome. From: Haematology

Care more so the client sings your praises.

Case Studies with Blood Cell Morphology and
Pathophysiology,

STYE

It could be an infection of sebaceous glands at the base of the
eyelashes or an infection of the sweat glands. It's not a
chronic condition, and usually disappears in one week
without treatment, or 4 days with antibiotics.

TRICHOTILLOMANIA

Is also known as hair pulling disorder is an impulse control
disorder characterized by the compulsive urge to pull out
ones own hair. If your client suffers from this disorder,
eyelash extensions are not a good solution.

TRICHOPHAGIA

Around a 15% of sufferers of trichotillomania eat their hair.
This is a serious psychological disorder, which could lead to
the complete loss of eyelashes and serious digestive
problems.

TRICHIASIS

In this condition the eyelashes are reversed positioned,
growing back to the ocular globe. Causes could be infections,
inflammations, autoimmune conditions, congenital defects,
and trauma (burns or injury).

It is important to know that at least 5% of clients may
develop an allergy to glue or the medical tape we use. Once

they develop this allergic reaction they are no longer a candidate for extensions and there is no known cure.

Google all eye disease photos and familiarise yourself with how they appear.

EYELASH TRANSPLANTS

In 2009, a team of British plastic surgeons performed the first eyelash transplant in UK. The micro-surgical procedure was conducted by Transform, the largest cosmetic surgery in UK.

It was the definitive solution for a problem of madarosis (loss of eyelashes) provoked by a trichotillomania disorder (obsessive compulsion of plucking one's hair) for Louise Thomas, a 19 year old teen from Stockport, Greater Manchester, who, after 17 years of suffering that disorder, she didn't have any eyelashes left.

The operation took approximately four hours and was done with local anaesthetic. It began by taking a hair graft from the back of the head, dissecting it under a microscope and placing it into tiny incisions in the eyelid, said Transform.

The patient paid a fee of approximately £3,500.-

This procedure is indicated for people who suffer of alopecia, trichotillomania or hair loss due to chemotherapy radiations.

Transplanted eyelashes usually thicken in four to six months after the surgery is done.

Shami Thomas, who carried out the operation, said that the procedure was both, safe and successful.

Actually the eyelash transplant is widely performed in US.

EYELASH GROWTH CYCLE.

Eyelashes are human hairs on the upper and lower eyelids that assist in the protection of the actual eye. Each eyelid has layers of eyelashes within a row. We usually have three to five layers of eyelashes, which protect and frame the eyes.

Eyelashes, have the similar anatomy of the human body hair. They are anchored to the eyelid by a root. There are small muscles located in the eyelids which, with a muscular contraction, -a reflexive and

automatic response-, they blink and close the eyelids before an external threat, such as particles of dust, or any foreign agent which could cause damages to the eyes.

In every blink the eyelashes close access to the eyes like curtains. In every blink, the eyes are irrigated with a lubricant secretion from sebaceous glands -tear glands- running along the edge of the eyelid, with their openings between the eyelashes. This lubrication ensures that the eyes don't dry out, keeping them wet and healthy. Unfortunately this does not happen with all humans.

Eyelashes on the upper eyelid are longer than those of the lower eyelid. The upper eyelashes can reach a length of an average of 12 mm., and tend to curve upwards. The upper eyelid has around seventy to one hundred and fifty lashes.

The lower eyelid has generally a row of sixty to one hundred eyelashes.

The lower lashes are usually thinner and curve downwards. This curved shape of both upper and lower eyelashes helps to slip sweat and foreign particles out of the eyes.

Like all the hair in the human body, eyelashes are a biological polymer, made up of about 10 per cent of water and 90 per cent of proteins, such as keratins, and melanin, the substances that give hair its colour.

Note: if you attach an extension to the early anagen lash the grafted lash will fall out within a week or so and you will have very unhappy clients.

Like all human hair, they are fed by follicles, located below the skin. In eyelashes, those follicles have also three phases of growth before an Exogen stage lash falls out: -

ANAGEN (GROWTH) PHASE:
The anagen phase is also called the growth phase. This is the phase when lashes, are actively growing, and it lasts between 30 and 45 days. Only about 40 percent of the upper lashes and 15 percent of the lower lashes are in the anagen phase at any one time. Each lash will grow to a specific length and then stop.

CATAGEN (TRANSITION) PHASE:
The catagen phase is also known as the transition phase. During this phase, the lash stops growing and the hair follicle shrinks. If an eyelash falls out or is plucked out during this phase, **it won't grow back right away** because the follicle needs to complete the catagen phase before it can move on to the next stage. This phase lasts between two and three weeks.

Care more so the client sings your praises.

Learn More to Earn More

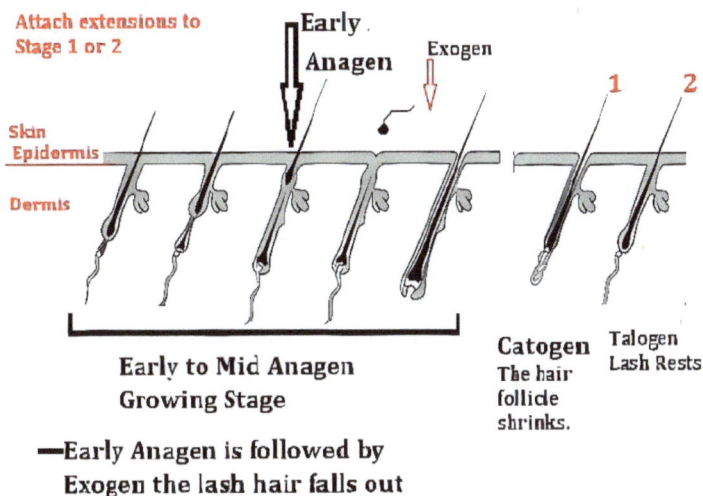

Attach extensions to Stage 1 or 2

Early Anagen

Exogen

1   2

Skin
Epidermis

Dermis

**Early to Mid Anagen
Growing Stage**

Catogen
The hair
follicle
shrinks.

Talogen
Lash Rests

—**Early Anagen is followed by
Exogen the lash hair falls out**

TELOGEN (RESTING) PHASE:

The telogen phase is also referred to as the resting phase.
This phase can last more than 100 days before the eyelash
falls out and a new one begins to grow. Because each
individual lash is in its own phase of the growing cycle, it's
normal for a few lashes to fall out most days. It typically
takes between four and eight weeks to fully replace an
eyelash.

EXOGEN FINAL

Exogen is when the hair eventually detaches and falls out.

It is best to attach to the Telogen lashes.

UNIQUE LASH VARIANCE

When an eyelash is pulled out or drops out, it needs about
two months to be regenerated.

You would now be thinking they are so close to each other and how do I know which lash is in mid anagen or talogen stage?

The longest of normal lashes are more than likely in the early anagen stage and have a new lash pushing the old lash out of the skin. Therefore, you would avoid these lashes

The natural lashes when given a good brush and comb will often remove lashes in the stage just after early anagen and approaching the exogen stage.

MAINTAINING HEALTHY SKIN AROUND THE EYES

Caring for the skin around the eyes is a delicate process. Because the skin around the eyes is much thinner, it not only tends to be the first place to show signs of aging, but also is more sensitive than the rest of the skin.

Therefore, extra care needs to be taken when choosing a skincare product for this area.

Products that contain gentle, non-irritating compounds that reduce the appearance of wrinkles (exfoliates), along with a wide range of vitamins, antioxidants, and skin-plumping substances are ideal choices.

When choosing products for the eye area, it is important that it be oil-free. Products containing oil increase the likelihood of clogged glands around the eyes that can lead to stye and other ocular problems. Unless it is a cold pressed based oil or an essential oil. It is when creams have an oil base that the problem arises.

However, an Aromatherapist knows the very best oils to use and prefer oils to creams.

Creams are usually loaded with preservatives. Although essential oils are named oils they are actually a liquid. Creams should never ever be used on the eyelid or eye lashes.

The unfortunate part of commercial oils based products that are not certified organic are - that they use cheap oils that have bleach in them.

All beauty treatment oils need to be a base oil that has been cold pressed and essential oils added, not fragrance oils.

EYE TREATMENT

My Favorite Aromatherapy Mix
In a clean, dark coloured, narrow neck bottle - pour 25 ml of cold pressed light Jojoba oil

Add:-
5 drops of Chamomile essential oil
 1 drop of Rose Geranium essential oils or   Rose oil if you can afford it.

Do not use fragrant oils.

This is one of the most healing and soothing eye oils anyone could ever use on their eyes. This mix would even cure eye mites.

On a freshly cleaned face in the evening just before you go to bed. Pat a few drops on the upper portion of the closed eyelids and just above the cheek bone. The eyes will draw the oils in so be sure not to apply too close to the lashes.

Use this mix every night for 1-2 weeks before having the eyelash extensions.

Remember that most eye specialist do not know a great deal about Aromatherapy products. Therefore, they give advice on shelf products. Some of the information here is also based on shelf products. All Beauty Therapists should consider taking part in Beauty School Books Aromatherapy Skincare Mixing Course.

Contact lens wearers in particular, should avoid products containing oil. The oil not only sticks to the lens causing blurred vision, but can also cause

permanent staining. To minimize the potential for contamination, people should avoid products packaged in a manner that requires "dipping" fingers into a jar.

The above oil should only be applied after removing the contact lenses in the evening.

Please refer to this site for more information
www.mediniche.com/ocularskincare.html

TRAIN YOUR CLIENT BROCHURE.

In your brochure train your client.

Add some useful information in your eye extension brochure. Personally I love a business card that folds like a card. When you give the client a card with her appointment date you should have a small leaflet on each service you offer and attach it to the card.

AFTERCARE DOS AND DON'TS

Do not cleanse eyes, shower, swim, use a steam or dry sauna for at least 24 hours after procedure, 24 hours is advised for proper bonding.
Avoid heat treatments like saunas and sun beds.
Always be gentle with lashes. Try not to sleep on them.
Do not use an eyelash curler.
Avoid all oil-based makeup products and eye-makeup remover.
Avoid waterproof mascara. There are mascaras on the market designed for eyelash extension, which I do retail.
Touch ups are recommended every 2-4 weeks
Get them removed by a professional
Never pick at them, if a lash is out of place cut it instead or brush them.
Brush eyelash extensions daily.

Eyelash Grafting and Party Lashes

Apply sealant to your lashes regularly following advice of the brand used.

CLEANING YOUR EYELASH EXTENSIONS

First thing within 24 hours use the saline we provided you with - to rinse your eyes. Cut the tip off the saline with clean scissors. Wash the scissors first, dry with a cotton pad and wipe with the alcohol wipe we have provided.

Ideally daily you should wash your eyelash extensions with shampoo. Mix Johnson and Johnson baby shampoo (or similar) with a little water and directly apply it to the lashes. Gently massage the lashes back and fore, then away from the eyelid. Daily allow the water from your shower to run over the eyelash extensions moving them sideways slightly with your little finger to get the water between the lashes.

Pat them dry with clear cottonwood pad.

Please remember your natural eyelashes (not extensions) fall out and another one grows back in the follicle to replace it, so don't panic if you lose a eyelash extensions while cleaning them. You would naturally lose 1 -5 lashes a day with or without eyelash extensions.

However, if you find you are losing a lot of eyelash extensions when you wash them, it could be that the eyelash extensions you have on are too long and not suited to your natural eyelash growth stage. Therefore the amount of eyelash extensions anchored to your natural lash isn't enough or they simply haven't been bonded correctly.

How to remove makeup around my eyelash extensions

After a day of wearing makeup you often find that makeup has gathered around the base of the eyelash extensions.

First clean your face in the way we have advised you.

Next dip a cotton tip into cleanser and work into the eye line nearest the eyelash root. Repeat this step with tip dipped in water, then spray the cotton tip with toner and work into the lash root line.

Never use the same cotton bud on both eyes as you may have an eye infection developing you are unaware of and pass it onto the other eye. You can always give your eyelashes a gentle brush at this stage being extremely careful not to damage the extensions.

EYELASH EXTENSIONS AND BLEPHARITIS

It is good practice to keep the eyelash extensions clean to prevent eyelash extension Blepharitis.

Blepharitis is when the hair follicle becomes infected and blocked. It becomes blocked with your skins natural oil called sebum, dead skin cells and bacteria, which hasn't been cleaned away. It basically looks like dandruff around your eyelash extensions. If you do find you have blepharitis it's best to ask your eyelash technician to remove the lashes and visit your GP for some topical ointment to apply to the eyelid to clean up the infection.

This isn't just for eyelash extensions wearers, this could easily happen to people who don't remove their mascara or generally clean their face daily.

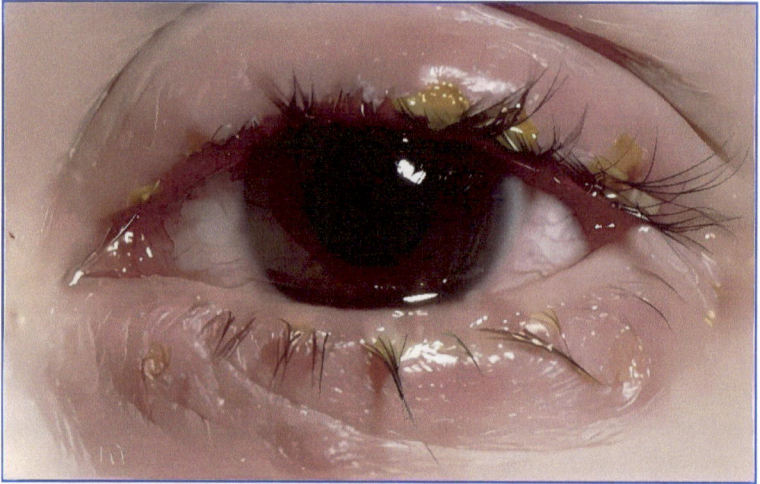

Blepharitis

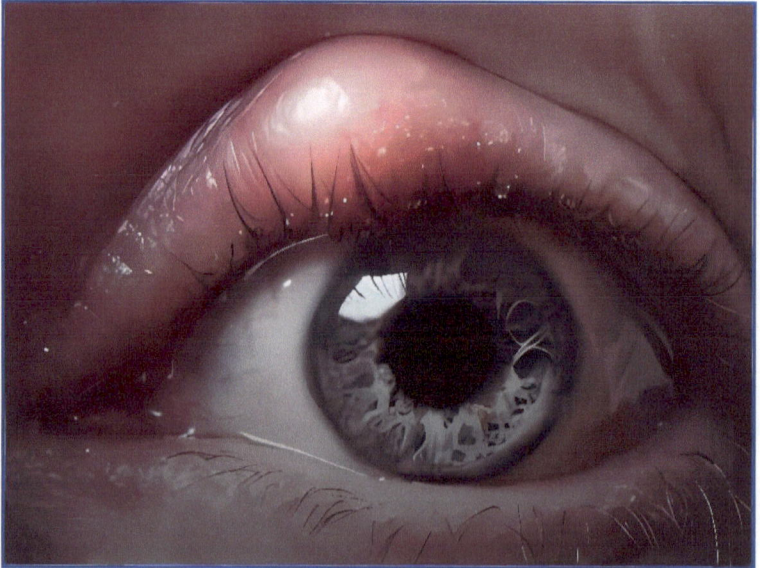

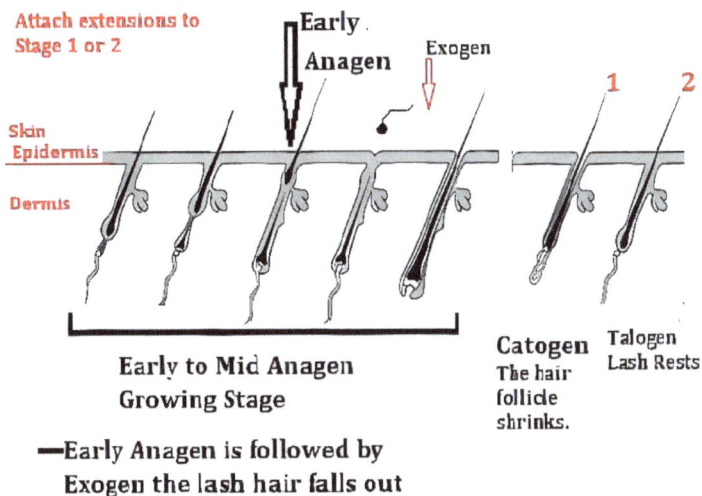

Attach extensions to Stage 1 or 2

Early Anagen

Exogen

1 2

Skin Epidermis

Dermis

Early to Mid Anagen Growing Stage

Catogen The hair follicle shrinks.

Talogen Lash Rests

—**Early Anagen is followed by Exogen the lash hair falls out**

Give the client these few photos with a brief explanation.

The above information is a good place to start. However, the more you as a therapist know about aftercare, the better equipped you will be - to advise your client.

A GOOD PLACE TO RESEARCH IS

https://visioneyeinstitute.com.au/eyematters/blepharitis/

WARNING

Never ever put eye lotions, creams nor oils on the lower lid section near the eyelash roots. The eye has a very strong pulse and will draw oils or creams into the eye. Treatments should be gently patted onto the upper section of the eye lid and slightly above the upper section of the bone structure found below the underside of the eye. So that means the bone around the eye cavity.

EYES DRAW CREAMS IN

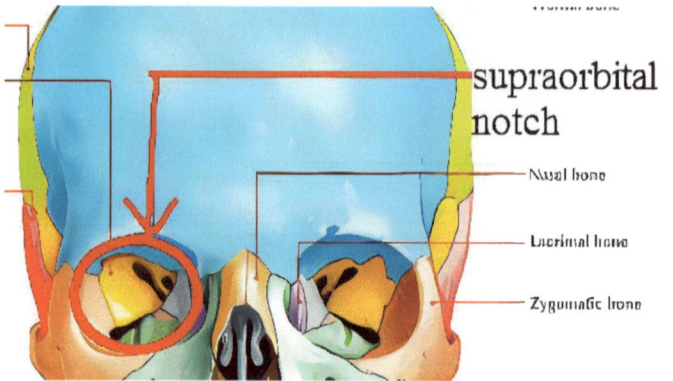

supraorbital notch

Nasal bone

Lacrimal bone

Zygomatic bone

Starting at the supraorbital foramen or the supraorbital process bone. Which is positioned, about a finger space below the eyebrow. It is a circular bone that also sits above the cheek bone. You can actually feel the hollow with your fingers.

Common skin exfoliates are alpha hydroxy acids, often referred to as AHA's. AHA's are a group of naturally occurring substances found in a variety of fruits, sugar cane and milk. They are not suitable for the delicate eye area.

They cause a loosening of the outer dead cell layers, which leads to exfoliation (sloughing of dead skin cells), thereby combating the build-up of corneocytes. The accelerated turnover allows the epidermis to become smoother and softer, and reduces the appearance of fine lines.

By thinning the dead cell layer, AHA's enhance the penetration of other important ingredients. AHA's also act as superb moisturizers due to their hydroscopic (water binding) ability. Only products containing a very mild AHA formula should be used on the delicate periocular area.

In addition to AHA's, other ingredients such as moisturizers, antioxidant vitamins and herbal extracts are important for caring for the skin around the eyes.

• Antioxidant Vitamins including Vitamins A, B-complex, C, D and beta-Carotene provide protection against free radical damage. Free radicals are "off balanced" microscopic molecules usually found in groups of thousands. They have the power to do extensive damage to the cell membrane as well as complete destruction to normal cells by robbing them of oxygen. Pollution, UV light, smoking, large quantities of alcohol and daily stress can trigger the production of free radicals. Antioxidants render free radicals harmless before they damage the skin's healthy cells.

• Moisturizers such as sodium hyaluronate help reduce fine lines caused by dehydration. Sodium

hyaluronate is the most effective humectant available, and has the ability to bind moisture in the amount of one thousand times its molecular weight.

• Herbal Extracts and Liposomes including chamomile, cornflower, bisabolol and lecithin decrease redness, puffiness and act to nourish, revitalize and rejuvenate the skin.

Notes:
Note 1. A vitamin capsule cut open and patted onto the skin. This gives fabulous results. You can use any oil based capsule.

Note 2. Cosmetic needling done by a Cosmetic tattooist will repair fine lines even deep lines will become barely noticeably. However, you will have unsightly red lines for about 6-12 days.

Note 3. A galvanic facial every week will lift the muscles in your face. You cannot give yourself a galvanic facial so you will need to barter for a good price with your beauty therapist. You should not

have galvanic facials until the face starts to drop around the age of thirty.

AROMATHERAPY SKINCARE

It has not been my intension in this book to explain skincare nor to explain Aromatherapy. I have written other books on these subjects.

Most of you would have done a module or two on Aromatherapy in beauty school while studying for you Certificate or Diploma in Beauty.

Ignorance is bliss but very dangerous when you step out of your comfort zone and into the world of the beauty business.

The more you learn the more you realize you do not know and should know. A Doctor would have studied skin during his/her training to become a GP but they do not profess to know and understand skin complaints. They give you a referral to a skin specialist.

Care more so the client sings your praises.

However, if it is a mild skin condition they will more than likely give you a prescription as a trial to see if the complaint subsides.

As an eyelash technician I feel you should at least understand that not everyone can afford to buy top shelf cosmetics. Therefore, you should be able to mix some product for those people. It has been proven that aromatherapy products make the very best difference on everyone skin.

Some of your clients wanting eyelash extensions have skin care issues and those should always be addressed.

Let say they want eyelash extensions but clearly have poorly cared for skin. It is your job to assist them in the preparation for the lashes.

When the eyelashes are extended their entire face becomes more open, with a lifted, younger, more youthful appearance. If their skin, is noticeably dry or dull that will be more noticeable as well. You need to advise them of this fact.

The Aromatherapy skincare mixing instructions below, although very basic instructions they have been designed for the novice mixer and are very safe blends even for a home user to mix and apply.

MAKING SKIN CARE

I have added a very small section on skincare mixing in this book. I feel that everyone will be well advised to mix their own skincare. I have produced other books on skincare mixing. However, this section will assist you to get started.

CLEANSERS

First check on what essential oils are safe for you to use. You may as well make a cleanser that is a cleanser as well as a healing agent.

Place 95 ml of olive oil into a 100 ml dark coloured narrow neck bottle.

You can use the bottle the cold pressed Olive oil comes in as it is usually a dark bottle. If you choose to use cooking oil that is fine as all olive oil is cold pressed and safe to use in cosmetic mixing. However, the bottle will probably be clear therefore - you will need to keep it in a brown paper bag.

Add 5-10 drops of your chosen essential oils.

Shake and you're done. Always return the lid to the bottles as soon as possible.
Store - in a cool dark cupboard.

After removing with soft tissues you will need to press the face and neck with a warm wet face cloth. Then rinse the cloth in warm water, wring it out and wipe the face with the warm wet cloth.

TONER

In a 100ml dark coloured narrow neck bottle place 95ml of cooled boiled water.
Add 5ml witch hazel
3 drops of essential oil.

Learn More to Earn More

The essential oils I use are 2 drops Rose Geranium and 1 drop of eucalyptus.

EYE MAKEUP REMOVER

Eye makeup remover for - stubborn eye makeup.

Place in a small plastic bottle 50ml baby oil and 3 drops of chamomile essential oil.

With your finger tips smooth gently a few drops onto a closed eye. Do one eye at a time.

Then rinse/ sponge off with a warm wet face cloth or sponge. Pat the skin dry and wipe over with cotton wool soaked in toner or a very mild astringent.

Baby oil is not a - healing oil it is a skin barrier. Do not use baby oil on any other part of your body it has been designed to stop urine penetrating the skin on baby's bottoms, vagina and penis.

Thus it will stop eye shadow and mascara from - penetrating the skin and assist these products to slide off the skin, during the cleaning process. The warm wet face cloth must be used to remove the oil from your eyes.

MOISTURIZER

Moisturizers are simple to make. Use a mix of base oils and 3 drops of essential oils. Pat onto skin 20 minutes before applying Makeup.

Also tone the skin before applying the moisturizer and again before applying makeup. A time lag between applying moisturizer and makeup should be approximately 20 minutes.

Good time management is to cleanse the face then moisturize. Go and do something else like make you bed or get dressed and have breakfast then apply your makeup.

Moisturizers take time to penetrate, unlike store bought products that have drying agents added to them.

All too often clients complain that they had their makeup done professionally for a special occasion and it did not last. They also say that the makeup seeped into their eyes and made their eyes watery. This is often due to the fact that their makeup was applied too soon after the moisturizer was applied. The other reason this can happen is the therapist or makeup artist applied the foundation makeup too close to the eyes. Eyes draw product in towards the eyeball that is why you should keep clear of the eye area. Cheap eyeliners and eye shadows will do the same.

Quality eye liners and eye shadows have been designed to set onto the skin and will not migrate into the eyes.

SKIN PEELS

Skin peels should be done at least once a month and never do them daily. They rid the body and face of dead skin cells. There are two very easy ways to give the skin a mini skin peel.

Rub your after sun body oil all over your body.

Place a capful of the oil into a small dish and add one tablespoon of ground sea salt.

Mix then rub this into your oiled body. Rub in a circular motion, as though you are trying to remove something.

Then have a long shower.

The other easy peel is to go to the beach and do the same as above but use the wet sand as your abrasive. I usually use coconut oil and sit on the water edge while I rub myself with the sand.

NIGHT CREAMS

Night Creams are far more complicated to mix. However, if you buy some coconut oil and add a few drops of Clary-sage and a few drops of Lavender plus

Rose oil you will have a night cream far superior to anything in the market place.

My favourite nigh oil is:

90 mill of olive oil
10 mill of wheat germ oil
2 drops Rose oil
6 drops Rose Geranium
2 drops Clary Sage

After sun

The best oil for after sun is 100ml Olive or Jojoba or Almond carrier oil to which you add 30 drops of Lavender and 5 drops of Lemon essential oils. Pour a little into your hand rub both hands together and work into your entire body.

 Note this mix is too strong for children and for your face so dilute it with Olive oil for your face and check children's mixing instructions in the section headed "A-Z of ailments" in my Aromatherapy books.

Bath Oils

Bath oils are easy to make and are the easiest way of nourishing the body inside and out. If mixed correctly they will assist with the healing process of all diseases/ailments of the mind, body and soul.

Refer to my section headed "A-Z of ailments" in my Aromatherapy books for a more informative list of mixing bath oils.

Mix 50 drops of Essential Oils in a dark glass bottle of 100 ml carrier oil.

Keep in a dark place never put on the window sill.

You can always Google what essentials are best for you. If you have no health conditions then you can use most of the safe oils.

Essential oils have a pulse. The odour molecules dance in the air. Incandescent lights can turn them into toxic odours. For this reason have a bath by candle light. Have the window and door closed in the bathroom so you can breathe in the aromatic healing odours.

MASKS

A mask is something that draws impurities out of the skin and acts as a tightening agent to assist with the ageing process. It further aids the skin from contamination, infectivity, corruptions and pollution. Pollutions in the air age the skin so a mask is a very important weekly skincare process.

Masks may be made from many products.

Sour cream
Sour cream or **plain yoghurt** may be applied to the skin and left to dry.

Lay in the body slant position for 10 minutes.
Then rinse/ sponge off with a warm wet face cloth or sponge. Pat the skin dry and wipe over with cottonwool soaked in toner or an astringent.
Egg White

Separate the white of an egg from the yoke whisk the egg white and apply to the skin.

Lay in the body slant position.

This will dry as stiff as a board so you do not want it to pull your skin in the wrong direction.

Then rinsed/ sponged off with a warm wet face cloth or sponge. Pat the skin dry and wipe over with cotton wool soaked in toner or an astringent.

Porridge or wheat biscuits.

Mix a little with a small quantity of warm water and apply to the skin.

Lay in the body slant position. This will dry as stiff as a board so you do not want it to pull your skin in the wrong direction.

Then rinse/ sponge off product from your face with a warm wet face cloth or sponge.

Pat the skin dry and wipe over with cotton wool soaked in toner or an astringent.

Clay,

Clay, Corn flour or fullers earth. Clay is by far the best. At the end of my organic skincare book you will find a page devoted to the use of clay. Fullers earth is not to be used on sensitive skin types. Purchased at Pharmacies/chemist shops or supermarket.

Clay may be purchased from beauticians. These days they like to call themselves Beauty Therapists or Beauty Salon/Clinics.

AROMATHERAPY EYE EXFOLIATE

In 50 ml of Grape seed cold pressed oil
Place 8 drops of Chamomile
5 drops of Rose oil or 3 drops Rose Geranium.
Plus 1 drop of Cary Sage

Store in a clean dark coloured bottle, This must be stored in a cool dark place (not in the refrigerator).

ONCE A WEEK.

Treat one eye at a time.

Place one teaspoon of this oil mixture, into a cup.

Mix with either 1/4 (quarter) teaspoon of corn flour or French white clay.

Gently massage onto the closed eye one eye at a time. Remove by splashing cool water onto the closed eye. Use your little finger when massaging the eyelids - as it has less strength in it then the other fingers.

Place a wet warm face cloth, onto the eye and complete the treatment by splashing cool water onto the eye and pat dry.

Repeat the treatment for the other eye.

French white clay used as a mask will also prevent the eyelids from sagging/drooping.

HEALTHY EYES

Tips for keeping the skin around the eyes healthy

In addition to choosing the proper skin care product, other things are important in maintaining healthy skin around the eyes:

Eye Drops that I so love that do not sting are "Systane" by Alcon Laboratories Australia Pty Limited Frenchs Forrest in NSW Australia. I use these on my dogs as well. They are so gentle.

• Drink plenty of water. Water plays a crucial role maintaining the elasticity of skin. But never more than 8 cups a day or there will be a condition that cases the heart to race and you will faint.

Excessive water consumption can cause exercise-associated hyponatremia, a potentially deadly condition where the body is unable to remove the water causing the sodium content of blood to be diluted to dangerously low levels.

• Avoid smoking cigarettes. Nicotine constricts blood vessels in the face and under the eyes. Constricted vessels also make it difficult for nutrients to be absorbed, which leads to a breakdown of collagen.

• Stay out of the sun. Overexposure to ultraviolet rays causes melanocytes, the pigment-producing cells, to mature abnormally. This results in age spots and uneven pigmentation. UV rays are responsible for up to 90% of aging and can add several years to your appearance.

• Wear sunglasses to avoid squinting.

• Get plenty of rest. Fatigue can cause skin to look pale and gaunt.

• Limit alcohol intake. Excessive drinking can cause dehydration, so limit yourself to a glass or two of wine every week

• Use cotton balls and olive oil when removing makeup to avoid unnecessary tugging on the delicate eyelid tissue. Olive oil is a great eye makeup remover so long as you completely remove with a hot compress.

• Use a quality professionally recommended skin care product for the area around the eyes. Preferable one that is made, by a local Aromatherapist.

By following the above information and choosing a skin care product with the right combination of ingredients will help keep the skin around your eyes looking younger.

To reduce the dark circles around your eyes, no matter what age you are, you must have at least six to eight hours sleep every night. Sleeping with your shoulders slightly elevated and head tilted towards the mattress would help you working against gravity; which causes fluid to collect in your lower eyelids resulting in dark circles.

Use an eye cream around the eyes to keep moisture in the skin. Better still, use the above eye moisturizer I have given you the recipe for.

When applying cream or make up around the eyes, use the ring finger (as it exerts less pressure). Never

ever on the actual eye lid. Remember the eye cavity bone is your guide to where the cosmetics end.

Don't rub eyes frequently as this can cause an eye infection and in turn causing infection in the skin around eyes. This is because; few of us bother to wash our hands before touching our eyes.

Eye care should not enter the eye area and must stop at the supraorbital bone.

AROMATHERAPY DO'S AND DON'TS:

DO'S:

Dip cotton-wool pads in chilled water or milk, lay in the beauty slant position and place on closed eyes for 10 minutes.

 A beauty Slant position means you lay down with a pillow under your shoulders. Your head must be tilted back towards the ground.

My favorite eye pad is Chamomile tea bags. Place two tea bags in hot water, take straight out and drain. When almost cool press out the water and place on your eyes for 10 minutes and please relax.

Rinse your eyes with warm water pat dry and apply eye oil not a cream to the upper lid. On the supraorbital bone

If a client complains that their eyes are tired after working all day with computers? Then grate a potato with its peel and apply on their closed eyelids for about 20 minutes they must relax completely. This is to prepare their eyes to have firm muscles. Then apply the chamomile tea bags to their eyes.

Sliced cucumber placed over your eyes will avoid developing dark circles.

Give a massage to the eyes, with your little finger by gentle finger movement

If their eyes are red or feeling itchy, massage their scalp with curd, to reduce the unwanted temperature around your eye skin. Also placing and ice pack wrapped in tissues works great.

Whenever possible they should wash their eyes with cold water. This will bring a sparkling feeling to your eye skin.

DON'T

Do not make a mixture for a client without checking essential oil contraindications against the client health conditions. You can view these on my website

TO REDUCE, PUFFY EYES.

Put two tablespoons in the freezer leave them in the freezer all the time. Each night apply the underside of the spoon to your eyes. Hold on your eyes for 5 minutes.

Always use cold pressed oils when mixing skin care. Always add essential oils to the cold pressed oils, **not fragrant oils**. Follow aromatherapy advice /recommendation for blending essential oils.

Essential oils **cannot** be used straight from the bottle onto your skin. They must be added to a base oil.

Read this entire section on my website
https://beautyschoolbooks.com.au/safety-chart/

Fish oil may also help ease dry eyes and age-related macular degeneration. Yogurt and cheese. "Both of these dairy products contain zinc, which is also beneficial for the eyes. Zinc is concentrated in the retina and helps vitamin A produce melanin, a pigment that helps protect the eyes.

AROMATHERAPY SAFE OILS

Always check blending instructions and contraindication for each essential oil. These chart can be viewed or purchased on our website https://beautyschoolbooks.com.au/safety-chart/

CYPRESS - Cypressus Sempervirens
Very popular with men, an excellent deodorant reduces both sweating & odour, plus fluid retention.

EUCALYPTUS - Eucalyptus Globulus
Need I explain this Australian oil? The aborigines believed the heat goes into the fire when they burn the leaves and the sickness goes out of the man/woman. It's a cure all.

FRANKINCENSE - Boswellia Carterii

A comforting resin. Used throughout the ages for ceremonies and ritual. Heals scar tissue, but can stupefy the brain in high doses or when used too often.

GARLIC - Allium Sativum
Antibiotic, also good oil for the heart and circulation.

GERANIUM - Pelargonium Graveoleus
Anti-depressant, uplifting, great for gall bladder, liver problems acne, broken capillaries.

GINGER - Zingiber Officinale
A body cleanser in childbirth that expels the placenta. A digestive aid, great for colic.

GRAPEFRUIT - Citrus Decumana
Uplifting and refreshing. High in vitamin C.

JASMINE - Jasminium grandiflorum
The concrete is mainly used in perfumery, used in China to treat Hepatitis. Aphrodisiac.

JUNIPER - Juniperus Communis **
Mainly used for cystitis and other urinary infections.

LAVENDER (TASMANIAN) - Lavendula Augustifolia
Burns heal almost instantly. The most popular and versatile essential oil. Relaxing, comforting and nurturing. Excellent oil for cancer patients. **Must not be used for people with low blood pressure. Nor Males during puberty as it has been documented to cause breast enlargements.**

LEMON - Citrus Limonum
Cooling, it is an excellent astringent for the skin, aids weight loss, arthritis & brittle nails.

But may decalcify bones if you or your clients calcium levels are low.
A Phototoxic oil.

LEMONGRASS - Cymbopogon Flexuosus
A sedative on the CNS and clears infections. a preservative. It can pose a significant risk of skin sensitization when used over 0.7% in topical applications. A little goes a very long way in topical formulations.

LIME - Citrus Aurantifolia
Used for dyspepsia, colds and fever.
Photosensitive oil. -only add to mixtures that you use on skin after dark.

MAY CHANG - Litsea Cubeba
Light and refreshing. A heart tonic for angina.
Maybe fatal if swallowed.

MARJORAM - Majorana Hortensis
Excellent for - all chest complaints. **Non toxic calming.**

MELISSA - Melissa Officinalis
Relaxing and relieving, helps dry up acne. Known as; lemon balm. Melissa softens extreme emotions, eases resentment, gladdens the heart and engages the soul find its own graceful rhythm. When making a skincare range use at 9% of usual dose.
Because this essential oil poses a higher risk of causing irritation and sensitization, it is recommended that it be avoided in the bath, even if it is solubilised/diluted.

MYRRH - Commiphora Molmol
Strengthening, a body preserver, great for weak gums ulcers and sores used in 1% dilution.

Care more so the client sings your praises.

Learn More to Earn More

Never to be taken internally.

NEROLI - Citrus Aurantium
Relaxing and soothing cardiac spasm and false angina.
Rejuvenates the skin.
Photosensitive.

ORANGE - Citrum Sinensis
Uplifting. Orange sets the mood for joyful communication.
Photosensitive.

PATCHOULI - Pogosernon Cablin
Grounding. Skin repair, nerve tonic, aphrodisiac.

ROSE OTTO -   Rosa Damascena
Nurturing and soothing. Rose is considered the "Queen" of
the essential oil kingdom. It is a nurturing tonic for the heart
and has excellent benefits for mature and sensitive skin.

ROSE GERANIUM
Similar to Geranium and by far my most favorite oil.
Excellent wound healer in both humans and animals.

SANDALWOOD - Santalum Album
Barbers rash, greasy or cracked skin. Encourages peace and
acceptance, excellent oil for meditation.

TEA TREE - Melaleuca Alternifolia
Active against all three infectious organisms: bacteria, fungi,
viruses. But please use with caution. It will also dry the skin
out to an unsightly dead look.

THYME - Thymus Serpyllurn Brilliant for muscles and
joints, oedema, obesity, sports injuries. Not good for people
with heart conditions.

The safest oils for skincare when untrained are Rose geranium, Clary sage, Lemon, Eucalyptus and Rose essential oils. I have had amazing results in animals and humans alike with Rose geranium.

Also in my book called the "Antique Healer". If you cannot get my book called the Antique Healer try to

find " Aromatherapy Know how". It is less expensive and has all the most important factors about mixing essential oils. It is However, a much smaller version.

.

DON'TS:

Don't wear contact lenses for extended periods of time nor overnight. This makes your eyes feel tired, hence giving unnecessary strain to your eye skin and eyes.

When you splash water, do not do this furiously believing doing this will take away tiredness instead wash gently as splashing may hurtle the smallest dust particles or an allergen which may damage the cornea which will again spoil your eye skin.

Don't use handkerchiefs to wipe eyes, instead use disposable tissues, which are more hygienic to your sensitive eye skin.

Don't sit near the television. View from a distance minimum of 15 feet/ 4 meters distance should be maintained from the television. keep your book at least two feet away to strengthen your eye skin muscles.

Use cream based eye makeup as powdery eye shadows can enter eyes that may cause irritation to the eye muscles and the skin nearby your eyes.

Care more so the client sings your praises.

Do not handle your eyes and eyelids in a harsh manner while using cleanses, as the skin will soon lose its strength by handling in a rough manner.

Don't use your mascara for more than a year, as it may weaken your eye skin. Give your eyes a break from mascara and eye shadow at least two days a week and always remove them quickly after work or an outing.

AROMATHERAPY CONTRA-INDICATIONS

Aromatic plant oils have general precautions associated with them. However, each client should be assessed before a blend is recommended.

The following factors are of particular importance when choosing blend ingredients.

A fresh mix made in a salon without preservatives is far more beneficial to your clients' skin than any products you purchase from skincare companies. Oils only last for two year so. Do not over stock and only buy from large companies that are selling thousands of bottles per day.

https://beautyschoolbooks.com.au/safety-chart/

IMPORTANT FACTORS

PREGNANCY

Certain oils should not be used during pregnancy as they can induce labour. When consulting with a female client you should find out if they are or they could be pregnant. Some clients may find this an intrusive or unusual question to be asked and you should explain why you are asking for this information. Don't assume that certain clients, for example teenagers or older women, could not be pregnant. If there is any doubt it is better to avoid those oils which should not be used during pregnancy. You should also consider your own safety when recommending blends and if you are, or could be, pregnant you should avoid working with those oils which can induce labour.

PHOTOTOXICITY

This is an excessive reaction to UV light caused by furanocoumarins (oxygen containing cyclic structures such as bergaptene) which are found in bergamot and the other citrus oils. In a phototoxic reaction the skin absorbs more UV light and produces abnormally dark areas of pigmentation and burning of the surrounding skin. Know as photosensitive. The pigmentation can last for years. When using phototoxic oils care should be taken with dilutions and clients should be advised to avoid exposure to the sun or UV lamps for a period of 12 to 24 hours after product application.

SENSITIZATION

Skin can react to certain oils with an allergic type of rash, blistering or redness. If the offending product is persistently used, contact dermatitis may occur.

CLIENT PREFERENCE

You should establish if there are any particular aromas that a client doesn't like. If you recommend a blend for its therapeutic properties it will not be beneficial if the client doesn't like the particular aromas.

PEPPERMINT - Mentha Piperita *
Clearing and refreshing a strong, sharp menthol aroma. **Not to be used on the face without an Aromatherapist consultation**. A small module added to your beauty therapy course does not make you an Aromatherapist.

PINE NEEDLE - Pinups Nigra
Not to be used in Aromatherapy. Gives great pleasure to a room, wonderful scents and clears away odd smells.

The international standard do not allow you nor I as an Aromatherapist, to administer or take essential oils orally/ingest nor add them to our food nor our drinks.

They can only be used as a topical application diluted in a base oil.

TRAY SETUP FOR PRACTICE.

The different size lashes,
One set of false eyelashes
Glue,
Glass or plastic square
Tweezers 2-3 types
Eyelash blowers
Eyelash curler
Paper towel
An orange or a practice doll
Q-Tips
Eyelash brush and comb
Tooth picks
Orange stick
Cotton wool pads
Gauge or callipers to measure the distance the glue is from the base of the false lashes
Tiny scissors
Eye was bowl and solution
Magnifying glasses

PRACTICE

1. Place the lashes on a doll or an orange. Use a hobby glue to stick them down.

2. Now set up your work tray as though you are going to work on a client.

3. Read the instruction above for applying lashes, named Procedure.

4. Watch the DVD that came with your kit several times.

Care more so the client sings your praises.

5. Remember the DVD is a video production so they have cut out mistakes the technician makes.

6. Now apply the grafted lashes to the false lashes.

7. Take a before, during and an after photo and send to your teacher.

8. Also take a photo of the amount of glue you are putting onto the lash.

9. It takes time to pick up speed and a practice session should be conducted daily until you are confident and fast.

10. Purchase a practice kit or a silicon practice block.

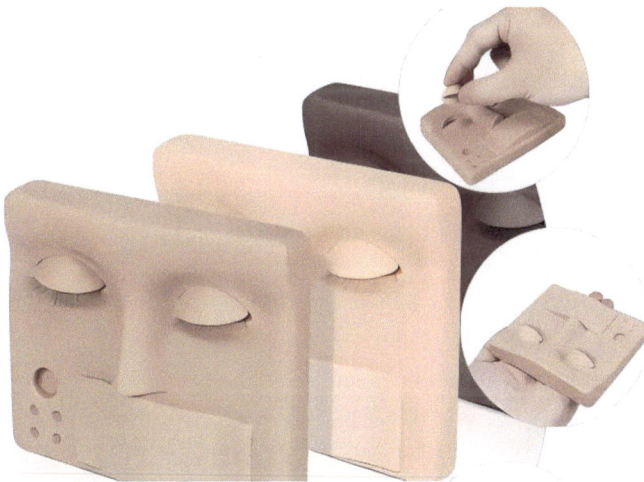

TEST THREE

EYELASH EXTENSION PRACTICE WITH TEACHER

You should have practiced at least five times before setting up an appointment with a teacher to watch you. Apply extension lashed on your doll.

If you do not have a teacher you can book a web conference training session with Robyna. Or Robyn. You will need Skype loaded onto your computer.

Email your details to beautyschoolbooks@gmail.com

Send your telephone numbers and Robyna or Robyn will call you if you live in Australia.

Internationals will need to correspond via email or Skype.

Set up a time with your teacher to watch you over video conference.

You will need to have a relative or close friend willing to have the extensions done.

You will also need to have a friend to hold the camera near the eyes of the client you are working on.

If you do not have a teacher it is still a good idea to film yourself doing your lashes on the doll and on the live person.

Watch these videos so you can view your mistakes.

Care more so the client sings your praises.

Learn More to Earn More

If the lashes are too long you can always trim them just a bit. Never trim too much or they will stick out. However, they will have a blunt unnatural shape and look unnatural.

ADVERTISE YOUR SERVICE.

Flyers are a great way to advertise your business. Have one in your shop window and do a letter box drop. I feel you young folk can make a better window advert better than I can.

Create a page or a group on Facebook, Instagram and Twitter. This social media places are where care instructions can live.
Make an eyelash and eyebrow care book and put on Google books as a down load.

Advertise on Gumtree, Facebook market place and eBay.

Give each client a card that gives then $10 off their next visit if they tell a friend about you. However, I found these cards are not required if you add extra client care to your services. People tell others about their excellent experience at your salon.

The best form of advertising is created by word of mouth. The more care you give your client the more likely they are to sing your praises.

TEST FOUR

Now make up a flyer and put up on the window of your shop.

If you are a mobile therapist make smaller versions and put up on notice boards.

Be sure you add your business name and telephone number to the flyer.

I would add a set of made up eyes to this poster. You can buy photos on the internet or take a lovely photo of a client and ask her permission in writing to use the photo.

TEST AFTERCARE INSTRUCTIONS

Within the next 24 hours...

Try not to cry or go out into the wind. Watery Eyes are salty and will dissolve the glue.

Care more so the client sings your praises.

Avoid oil-based cleansers, lotion or eye makeup removers. These products will dissolve the eyelash bonding agent. Instead, use plain water or water-based gel cleansers or aromatherapy cleansers with a gel base.

You may wish to use a Q-tip to gently remove eye makeup around the lash line.

We have provided you with mascara style brushed and they can be used daily to gently brush your lashes.

For stubborn makeup that may have become lodged in the eyelashes place a small quantity of baby shampoo on a mascara brush and roll onto the lashes. Rinse well with warm water. Do one eye at at time so you can keep the eyes closed.

Do not use waterproof mascara. The ingredients in this type of mascara will dissolve the bonding agent and your lashes will fall off when you take the mascara off.

If you feel you must wear mascara... apply only" water-based" mascara on your lash tips, not at the base of your lashes. Application at the lash base may break the lash and/or create a clump of mascara in your lash line.

Again, most women do not feel the need to apply any mascara at all. If you accidentally drop some powder on your lashes, simply remove with a Q-tip moistened in plain water in order for your dark lashes to reappear again.

Avoid using a mechanical eyelash curler. Instead, use a heated eyelash curler sparingly. Prolonged heat to the lashes may cause them to come loose as it will weaken the glues bond.

Schedule a "touch-up" procedure in 3-4 weeks. "Touch-ups" or "infill" are highly recommended in order to maintain a full, lush lash line. I swim every day and have to get my face under the shower with water pelting onto my face. I love the water. Therefore, I need my infill done every three weeks.

Some of my clients come every six weeks others every eight weeks. Should the lashes become annoying then take them off and give lashes a break for a few weeks.

First apply a warm compress to the lashes to break the glue bond.

Pat dry.

You can remove them by gently rubbing with olive oil mixed with ground sea salt. Mix 2 tablespoons olive oil with quarter teaspoon of ground salt. Bush onto eyelashes then use your fingers to rub the lashes without rubbing the eye shin.

Then apply a warm compress or book in to have the salon staff remove them for you.

You should have an infill done every two- three weeks.

The test number five requires you to improve on this aftercare and submit to your teacher.

TEST FIVE

AFTERCARE INSTRUCTIONS

Make up an aftercare sheet with your salon details and email to your teacher.

TEST SIX WRITTEN EXAM

Question:-
TYPICAL EYELASH EXTENSION EXAM QUESTIONS

1. How long do eyelash extensions last?
 a. One week.
 b. Four weeks.
 c. Depends on your lash cycle.
 d. They last forever.

2. Can you apply mascara to your extension /volume lash extensions?
a. No. It is not recommended to apply mascara to extension /volume lashes.
b. Yes, any kind.
c. Yes, it is recommended to wear mascara every day.
d. Yes, water-based mascaras only.

3. How often should you cleanse your lashes?
 a. Every day.
 b. Never.
 c. Once a week.
 d. Twice a week.

e. We recommend you clean your extensions at least 2 – 3 times a week. However, if you want to keep your lashes super fresh and fluffy you should clean them every day especially if you wear eye makeup or have oily skin. But, never on the day of or the day after the extensions are applied.

4. Which situation may cause damage to your natural lash?
a. Using Cyanoacrylate in your adhesive.
b. Sealing the lashes after application.
c. Using blunt tweezers.
d. Attaching one extension to multiple natural lashes.

5. Which lash extension will shed first.
a. The extension placed on the anagen lash.
b. The extension placed on the catagen lash.
c. The extension placed on the telogen lash.
d. They should all shed at the same rate.

6. Traction Alopecia is caused by:
a. An auto-immune disease.
b. A bacterial infection
c. A pulling force being applied to the natural lash.
d. Blepharitis.

7. It is not recommended to use the following lash diameter for extensions.
a. .05
b. .07
c. .10
d. .20

8. Which curl is the most popular for extension
a. J-Curl

b. B-Curl
c. C-Curl
d. D-Curl

9. Which element causes extension glue to weaken instantly?
a. Tears
b. Water.

10. What method do you use to disinfect your tweezers?
a. Acetone.
b. Hospital grade disinfectant.
c. 90% alcohol.
d. They should be scrubbed with green soap under running water.
e. They need to be autoclaved after scrubbing at a scrub sink with green soap.

11. True or False. It is important to perform a patch test on every client prior to applying a full set.
Your clients can develop an allergy to adhesives even if they have been receiving lash services for a long period of time without difficulties.
12. True or False Blepharitis is a common eye disorder that results in inflammation of the eyelids, causing red, irritated, itchy eyes, and the formation of dandruff like scales.
13. True or False It is typical for up to 5% of your clients to develop an allergy or sensitivity to lash adhesive at some time.
14. True or False I can reuse my tools after cleaning them with hospital grade disinfectant
15. True or False Wearing contact lenses during a procedure will cause problems
16. True or False. Post-Care includes giving your client after-care instructions

17. True or False. Your clients can develop an allergy to adhesives even if they have been receiving lash services for a long period of time without difficulties

18. True or False. You should paint the natural lash with adhesive prior to placing your extension

19. True or False. It is safe to apply up to 10 fine extensions onto one natural lash.

When Appling Extension ?

a. **Apply to one eye until all 25 to 30 lashes' have been applied**

b. **Apply 3 to 4 lashes on one eye then on the other eye**

EXAM ANSWERS

The answers have been placed on our website.
After answering the above questions you may check your answers at:-

https://beautyschoolbooks.com.au/eyelash-eyebrow-extensions/

PARTY LASHES

WHAT ARE PARTY LASHES?

Party lashes can be a row of lashes called "False Eyelashes" or Bunches of Lashes.

BUNCHES OF LASHES

Bunches of lashes know as party lashes. Smaller bunches are also called extension / volume   lashes. You are able to purchase in 2D to 5D and Hollywood volume. 2D has two lashes and 5D has 5 lashes in the bunch.

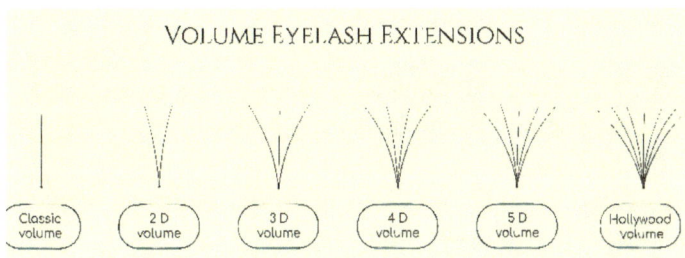

VOLUME EYELASH EXTENSIONS

Classic volume • 2 D volume • 3 D volume • 4 D volume • 5 D volume • Hollywood volume

Bunches of lashes are groups of lashes bonded together. You can just place a few at the outside edge of your natural lashes or place a full or half a row of them on your natural lashes. When glued 1 mm above the root of the natural lash onto the natural lash, they will last for two to four weeks.
This will naturally depend on several conditions.

THE GLUE IRRITATION

The less glue that is used is the best. Too much glue will cause irritation to the eyes and cause the natural lashes to droop and become very heavy. The glue sets hard and becomes very prickly/sharp and will pierce the soft tissues around the eyes. This causes an uncomfortable situation and the person will want to constantly rub their eyes. When their lashes droop they can see a dark shadow and this will cause them to push the lashes up out of their line of sight.

When you dip the end of the lash in the glue, wipe off the excess on a piece of foil or a plastic/glass dish.

The quality of the glue is vital. Never ever put glue into the refrigerator. Glue should be tossed into the bin after a few months and new glue purchased.

You will know when it is time to dispose of the glue when it is hard to coat the end of the lash with the glue.

Attach extension to the natural lashes about 2- 3mm above natural lash root, not on the skin.

When you attach a couple of lashes use a tooth pick to roll off the excess glue from the underside of the lashes. The toothpick should only be used once then a new one used on the next few lashes. I actually do this with every lash as I place onto the natural lashes.

FALSE LASHES

False lashes are usually a string of lashes. The type of glue used is designed for them to stay on for just a few hours. This service can be offered at the salon or you can sell them over the counter to customer. They come in a variety of thicknesses and shapes.

With all false, part and grafted lashes the glue and lashes should be glued to the natural lash not the skin.

 Bunches of lashes and false lashes come in a multitude of lengths and styles.

Some have feathers on the outer edge and some have diamonds on the tips of the lashes. They can be flirty, natural looking or extreme.

The reason we call them party lashes is because they are intended for a party. They will usually only stay on for a few hours to a few days. They are glued on the natural lashes close to the root of the natural lash.

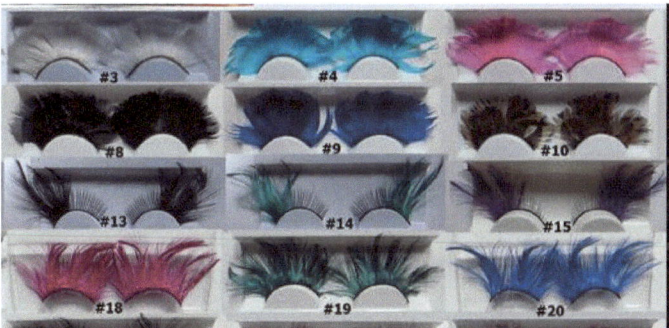

Rows of false lashes

A variety of these is a must have in your kit. You hold one row on the clients eye, just one of her eyes.

This way both you and her - can decide what type of lashes to apply and the shape.

I have found eBay has an endless supply of party lashes. Type " False lashes" into their search engine {bar} and you will be pleasantly surprised. The above photo shows several different types of false lash sets and you would find this helpful as a single use false lash to hold on the clients eyes. Do this while she decides which type of extensions she would enjoy and while you are conducting a consultation for grafted lashes. Plus there is a good variety for when applying false lashes for that special occasion.

EYELASH EDUCATION

People need to be informed on how to care for their lashes and cleaning of their face.

You need to have experienced both types of lashes using a few different glues before you can fully understand how to write up an education sheet for a client. The education sheet should be on the back of the aftercare sheet.

Party lashes are designed to last a few hours. However, with the way we have applied them for you, you should be able to get a week or more from your lovely lashes. For Party lashes to last 1-3 days, it is best to wash your face with cold or cool water.

It is best not to dive into a swimming pool or the ocean. Just walk in and keep your head above water.

Best not to get your lashes wet for 12 hours after they have been attached.

Best not to wear too much eye makeup that needs removing with oil based cleanser.

Try not to rub your eyes.

Try not to cry. Tears contain Over 1500 proteins, including lactoferrin, lipocalin, and IgA that will dissolve the glue

Try not to get your foundation or powder onto the lashes.

Do not apply mascara unless you are happy for them <u>not</u> to last.

Return to the salon before they are too thin. In other words if you are going somewhere on Saturday try to

have an infill done on Thursday or Friday or best still on the Saturday. If we are applying party lashes or false eyelashes then it is best to have them applied just hours before the event.

For grafted lashes- If your eyelashes still look great after two weeks make an appointment to have an infill in the beginning of the third week.

For false eyelashes they should be removed and reapplied. I try never to go for four weeks before having my infill. That way my lashes always look great.

These instructions apply to both party/false and grafted lashes. However, grafted lashes will definitely last longer than party lashes and have been designed that way.

Grafted lashes look more natural and will stay on longer because they are lighter and are attached one by one above the root to the tip of each of your own personal lashes.

Here I would add a good close up shot of each type of lash service you offer in your salon.

Students by incorporating an education and an after care sheet to suit both types of lashes is the smart option.

It serves you in several ways.

Less forms to worry about

You'll be less inclined to give out the wrong instruction sheet.

It informs the client about both services.

Sky Extension glue with the bluecap has had some good write ups . Google the ingredients lists of this glue company. I did and was impressed. But your clients will know which glue suits them best. Do some testing on family and friends.

Never ever keep any glue in the refrigerator.

The quality of the glue is vital.

Glue should be tossed into the bin after a few months and new glue purchased. You will know when it is time to

Care more so the client sings your praises.

dispose of the glue when it is hard to coat the end of the lash with the glue.

When you performing grafted lashes you attach a couple of lashes then use a tooth pick to roll off the excess glue from the underside of the lashes. The toothpick should only be used once then a new one used on the next few lashes. I actually do this with every bunch I place on the lashes.

When attaching false strings of lashed see below how to add glue to the lashes.
Inhaling the fumes from lash adhesive can have serious effects on you and your clients' health.

That's why this article will cover health issues from lash adhesives and what you can do to protect yourself.

WHAT INGREDIENTS ARE IN EYELASH EXTENSION GLUE?
Lash adhesive is made up of a bunch of different chemicals. Two of those chemicals can have serious impacts on our health.

The first chemical is called cyanoacrylate. This class of compounds is used for quick-setting adhesives. Your lash adhesive sets in 1 second BECAUSE it's got cyanoacrylate in it.

Formaldehyde isn't in the lash adhesive itself, but it is released when your glue dries. That being said, even if your glue advertises itself as "formaldehyde-free," you're not safe. Companies like to say their products are formaldehyde-free because it makes it seem healthier, but really, any lash glue that has cyanoacrylate in it (which is all of them right now) will release formaldehyde when it hardens.

So even though your lash adhesive might be formaldehyde-free, you're still prone to all of the side effects.

WHAT ARE SIDE EFFECTS OF EYELASH EXTENSION GLUE?

Cyanoacrylate may be our lash setting secret weapon, but it's got some nasty impacts, too:

I.   It can irritate your respiratory tract (eyes, nose, throat, lungs).

II.   It can cause an allergic reaction if it touches your skin.

III. It can cause flu-like symptoms (exhaustion, stuffy nose, sluggishness, etc).

IV.   It can cause dry or itchy eyes.

V.   It can cause headaches or light headedness.

VI.   It can cause nausea.

VII. It can make it hard for you to breathe.

HOW TO KEEP YOURSELF SAFE FROM LASH ADHESIVES

Now that you know your lash glue may be causing side effects, here's what you can do to protect yourself:

1: YOUR MASK
Your paper mask isn't protecting you or your client from anything but your bad breath.

Only a mask with a carbon filter can truly protect you. Masks recommended include a VOC gas or vapor mask. Change out the filter in your mask every 3-4 clients and keep your filter cartridges in the fridge to help them last longer.

The recommended one is the 3M Rugged Comfort Half Facepiece Reusable Respirator with the 3M 6000 Series Gas/Vapour Respirator Cartridges.

2: LET THE AIR FLOW
Make sure your workspace is open and airy. Not only will that help you breathe more safely, it'll look great, too! ;)

After each client, open the doors and windows to your studio to air out the fumes. Use an air purifier with a carbon filter to keep the air within your space as healthy as possible

If you've got the cash, get a fume extraction system. Your lungs will thank you! A recommend one is the Whisper Salon Source Capture System for Lash Artists.

Applying Glue to Strip Lashes

First used tweezers to gently remove the lash from the pack.

Hold the lash to your clients eye and take a good look at the length and the shape. Do the same if you are applying the lashes to yourself.

Next trim the lash to suite your eyes length and shape.

Trim from the outer corner where the longer lashes are. Do not trim the inner corner or they will not graduate in shape and will look very artificial.

Do not apply too close to the inner corner or the lashes will feel like they are stabbing you during the day.

Do not curl the natural lashes as they say to do in some of the instructions in the pack. This will make the placement of the false lashes almost impossible.

You do not want the lash base to extend all the way to the outer edge of your eye they will make you look tired.

For a mature age person it is better that the lashes are longer in the middle. This will make the eyes appear more wide open, and take the focus off the crows feet.
The thick lash effect is for younger people.

Care more so the client sings your praises.

Learn More to Earn More

Apply glue to a stick. This will save money on brushes and save cleanup time. Next slide the lash along the stick.

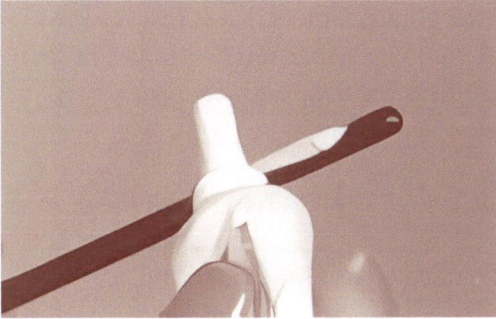

Next carefully and with a light pressure, slide the lash along the stick. Try not to get too much glue on the lashes. Base line.

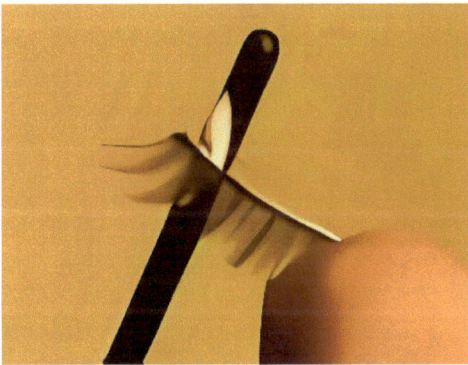

Next - Then slide the lash along the stick where there is no glue to smooth out the glue line and remove excess glue.

Sit the eyelash down on a dish for a minute or two so the glue sets a little before you apply. Be sure to sit them upside down so the glue does not touch the dish.

Look down into a magnifying mirror.

Then drop the lash onto your natural lashes.

Next wait a minute so the glue is almost dry. Then squeeze your natural lashes and the false lashes together. Start in the middle, then inner edge near the nose and work your way along the lashes.

Use a light pressure you do not want to remove all the glue.

Use black glue not a clear, as clear glue turns whitish when dry.

When they are both in place, run a line of black eyeliner along the joint. Liquid eyeliner is best.

Next very gently run mascara under the natural lashes to blend the colour of the false lashes and your natural lashes.

 Watch this video.
https://www.youtube.com/watch?v=-jigicP1Qvo

The only thing I disagree with she adds the glue to the lashes. It is best to apply the glue to an orange stick or chop stick (must be a wooden one).

Then run the false lash along the stick and then run along the other end of the stick to remove the excess glue.

You will love her very bright bubbly personality. More to the point she gives an excellent tutorial. I watched

twenty videos before choosing which one to recommend to you my faithful readers.

Care more so the client sings your praises.

PARTY LASHES, VERSES GRAFTED LASHES.

Grafted lashes look very natural. They last for several weeks. Party lashes last from a few hours to a few days.

You can also add mascara and dive into a pool or the ocean when you have Grafted Lashes.

Grafted lashes take 1 hour to 2 hours to apply. Party lashes take 10 – 15 minutes to apply.

Grafted Lashes cost from $100 to $250 to have applied.

Party lashes cost $20 to $75 to have applied.

The glue for grafted lashes costs $76 the glue for Party lashes cost about $12. Both glues will be used for at least 6 sets of lashes.

However, both glues must be used within two months.

WATCH YOU TUBE VIDEO

Many years ago this was the best video I could find. Now days there are better ones to watch but it is well worth your time.

http://www.youtube.com/watch?v=e-acf94MOxk&feature=related

GRAFTED EYELASH KIT

4 Jars of Mink Lashes
1 Jar Eyelash Cleaner
Eyelash Brush
2 Sets of Tweezers
1 Air Pump to dry lashes
1 Jar of glue
1 Jar of eyelash remover.
1 Roll of tape to protect lower lashes
1 set of practice lashes

You will also need:-
Cottonwool pads good quality.

Cotton tips
Paper towel
Dental chain
Beauty Bed
2 large towels. 1 goes under client 1 on top of client.
2 large hand towels. One goes around her feet. One around her neck secured with the dental chain

Care more so the client sings your praises.   Page | 152

2 pillows. One goes under their shoulders and one under their knees.
A good quality cleanser
A good quality toner.

Buy a few more sets of tweezers as the ones in the kit do not suit everyone.

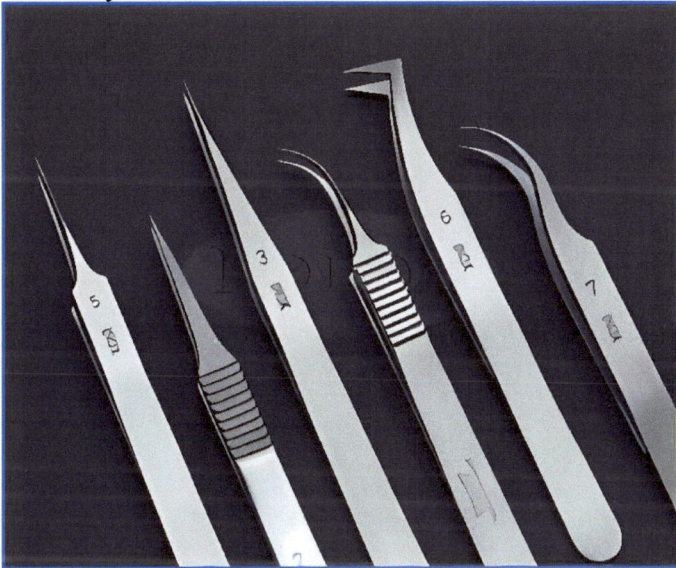

Titanium are best as you can autoclave them.
If you can afford a doll we recommend you buy one from a hairdressing supplier. It is great to have a doll on display with one eye done with party lashes and one with eyelash grating in your shop window. Add a sign to sit in front of the doll. It draws in business.

A Typical Eyelash Extension Kit

1st Allow me to explain the eyelashes come in jars with hundreds in each jar. Some come attached to a piece of cardboard.

They come in a few shapes the most popular shapes are - a "J" shape and a "C" shape

They come in 2-3 thicknesses

They come in several colours.

Usually Black, Brown, Blue, Purple, Green and Red,

Suppliers usually just send Black Lashes. If you want other colours, you need to specify what you want to the supplier..

LARGE KIT

A large Kit is not necessary for you to start off with. But this is what would come in a large kit.

3 Premium eyelash 0.15mm diameters, each 1 case (1gram) of 8 mm / 10 mm /12mm

3 Premium eyelash 0.20mm diameters, each 1 case (1gram) of 8mm / 10mm / 12mm

3 Premium coloured eyelash 0.15mm diameter, blue/purple/pink, each 1 case (1gram)

Glue black 1 bottle (sensitive) 10ml,

Glue black 1 bottle (very strong) 10ml,

Glue Remover high grade 1 bottle 10ml,

1 Extension /volume -up Mascara

3 Sets of tweezers curved type to select real lash for extension 3 pieces, Straight type to spread glue on lash. However, I use an orange stick for this.

Heated eyelash curler

Mini handy mirror 1 pc,

Good quality Irish diamond circle type for glue base

2 Good quality rubber sponge to clean around eyes,

Mini scissors for eyelash 1 pc,

Handy type rubber air-blower 1 pc,

False eyelashes for practice 1 pair,

Medical adhesive tape for application work,

Comb-brush for eyelash 1 pc,

1 Eyelash curler

1 Beauty Case 275mm(L) x 165mm(W) x 195mm(H)

Note: Unless you are going to be doing a lot of eyelash extensions this kit is too expensive. The glue does go off after about six month- one year. Buy a kit with only one bottle of glue.

If you do your work correctly there will be no sting to the eyes from the glue. The glue becomes a problem if you get it on the skin or in their eyes.

Place it too close to the skin at the lash root or if you use too much. Check the "Tray setup" section for other items you will require.

SMALL KIT CONTAINS:-

1 Premium eyelash 0.15 mm diameter, each 1 case (1 gram) of 8 mm/10 mm /12 mm
1 Premium eyelash 0.20 mm diameter, each 1 case (1 gram) of 8 mm / 10 mm /12 mm
1 Glue black 1 bottle (sensitive) 10 ml,
Glue Remover high grade 1 bottle.
Tweezers Curved type to select real lash for extension 3 pieces, Straight type to pick up extension lash.
Good quality rubber sponge to clean around eyes. You will need lots as these are single use.
Mini scissors for eyelash 1 pc,
Handy type rubber air-blower 1 pc,
False eyelashes for practice 1 pair ,
Medical adhesive tape for application work
Comb-brush for eyelash 1 pc,
Beauty Case 275 mm(L) x 165 mm(W) x 195 mm(H) 1 pc

Note: You usually find that the tweezers that come in the kit do not squeeze together well enough to do the picking up of the lash. You will need to try several types of tweezers until you get the set that suits you. Also they are not surgical steel and cannot be autoclaved. Therefore, you need to add a little plastic wrap to the tips to prevent cross contamination.

Care more so the client sings your praises.

Learn More to Earn More

It is best to buy medical grade tweezers so they can be sterilized.

HEALTH AND SAFETY

As an eyelash - technicians, it is important to know all health and safety regulations.

All items used must either be single use or surgical steel so they can be scrubbed in a separate scrub sink and autoclaved.

Therefore, tweezers must be of 1st grade quality.
Any item or tool that touches the skin is to be autoclaved after each use or thrown away.

The treatment room and bed must be completely cleaned after each use. Tweezers must not be coloured.

The facts sheets can be found at this web address

https://www.health.nsw.gov.au/environment/factsheets/Pages/beauty-treatment.aspx

or Google:-
Health and safety for the beauty room.
Skin penetration for beauty rooms
Infection control for the beauty room

Tweezers I prefer Titanium
Titanium tweezers do not shed particles like stainless steel tweezers. Titanium is light weight, high strength, non-magnetic material. Titanium causes less skin reactions.

DEAR STUDENT

Allow me to share with you what happens to me during an eyelash extension, procedure.

A truly peaceful emotion centres my being. A feeling of utopia unfolds as I watch the process enhancing the face of a client. It is an amazing joyous feeling. It is exciting. That's why clients can become addicted to

having their eyelashes extended. It is a lovely feminine course of action. and for a client having beautiful eyelashes can become addictive. Giving them an emotional lift will flow onto you.

Therefore you need to do it right so they can continue to feel like a very pretty woman. Do not turn this into a burden for them.

For over fifty years I was working in hairdressing and beauty salons. During this time I have trained many people to apply eyelashes. They were very popular in the 1950 and are still very popular today. To add to my credits I was chosen to write both the Australian and the international beauty industry assessment and training programs for the Government Standards Association.

Eyelash extensions lift the entire face giving it a more youthful appearance. If you gain 10% of the joy that I have experienced - you will be a very happy person and love your work. If you slap the eyelashes on causing eye problems and

Care more so the client sings your praises.

eyelashes to fall out quickly you will have complaining clients and that turns your day into a nightmare.

For you to become an expert and gain a good reputation - as a professional. You must understand the basics of eye anatomy, eyelash diseases and most importantly the natural eyelash type to attach eyelashes to.

We cannot cover all you need to know here in this course. Most of you will have already studied skin science and anatomy.

However, we have supplied you with enough information to tease your appetite for knowledge. It is imperative to research your new skills. And more so to practice the use of your tools so you can gain speed.

Watch the videos we have recommended in this manual before you begin and again every few months to refresh your knowledge.

At Beauty School Books Distance Learning Academe we strive to produce experts. The more you learn about your new skill, the more professional you will become.

The quicker you become a professional the better. Practice many times as per the practice instructions before you begin practicing on humans.

Before you begin eyelash extension it is important to note that, to gain insurance you will be expected to

have completed other forms of beauty therapy training.

WRBCS409A - Apply knowledge of skin science to beauty therapy treatments. Which is part of the WRB04 Beauty

Eyelash Grafting and Party Lashes

Training Package. Superseded by **SIBBCCS404A - Work in a skin therapies framework**
https://training.gov.au/Training/Details/SIBBCCS404A

It is a core unit for the following qualifications:

- WRB40104 Certificate IV in Beauty Therapy
- WRB50104 Diploma of Beauty Therapy

The guide has been designed to help you develop the skills and knowledge required to apply the principles of eyelash grafting to beauty therapy treatments. We expect you have a good knowledge of:

How to apply knowledge of skin science to beauty therapy treatments

6. Apply knowledge of skin disorders to beauty therapy treatments.

7. Promote skin health and care.

8. Know and understand eyelash growth cycle.

9. Know which eyelash to attach the grafted lash to.

10. Check that you have extremely good eyesight.

11. Without these elements of competency you should not be considering eyelash extensions as a trade.

Identifying how the skin grows and develops as well as changes that affect the skin over time, will help you to develop an under-standing of the affects of a range of different beauty therapy treatments and the techniques that are applied in the performance of these treatments.

For example facial treatments for mature skin may make use of products and techniques that are different than we use for

Care more so the client sings your praises.   Page | 160

a younger skin. Similarly different massage techniques would probably be used on a more mature skin compared to a younger skin.

CERTIFICATE COURSE

We only offer video sessions for the training. If you have a beauty therapist or school nearby you are best to do the training session with them. After you have worked through this eyelash training manual watched some YouTube videos and practiced f you would like do a certificate course

Contact:-
Beauty School Books
http://www.beautyschoolbooks.com.au

Email mailto:beautyschoolbooks@gmail.com

Beauty School Books site will soon be loaded with how to pages on all:-

Beauty tips
Beauty books
Body Piercing
Hair Styles
Dreadlocks
Fashion Tips And More
Forms for your business can be purchased.

REQUIRED SKILLS AND KNOWLEDGE

The following knowledge must be assessed as part of this unit: relevant health and hygiene regulations relevant occupational health and safety regulations and requirements infection control procedures and the application of universal precautions appearance of common skin types and conditions, including:
- Normal, dry, oily or combination
- Sensitive
- Pigmented
- Couperose
- Damaged
- Mature appearance of contraindications and adverse effects when applying false eyelashes following in regard to make-up services:
- Facial shapes and their relationship to the elements and principles of design
- Effects of natural and artificial light on cosmetics
- colour design principles
- colour wheel
- Primary, secondary, complementary colours, and grey scale
- tonal value, hue and shade cosmetic ingredients in relevant make-up products, particularly in regard to their likely effects on the skin effect of changes created by specific make-up products and colour application techniques workplace skin care and make-up product range effects and benefits of a defined range of workplace skin care and make-up products. Client care is always your best tool to success. Your clients tell their friends and their friends tell their friends that you are a cut about the rest.

Most clients hop around to different salons for treatments and will know the difference between a competent and incompetent, bungling, unskilled therapist.

To learn the skill to work on yourself and family is great but to learn to work on paying clients is a totally different

DEAR HOME USER,

Hi, if you are considering applying eyelash extensions at home you will find the step by step instructions useful. However, we suggest you have your first set done by a qualified eyelash technician. Then perhaps have an instruction lesson from your Beauty Therapist on how to do your infill. The only problem you will have is the cost of the fixative (glue) it is very expensive and as you may not be using it very often then it may go off before you get your money's worth. Retail it's about $75.AU

There are cheaper versions to be found on the internet However, we recommend you check the ingredient list before you purchase the glue. We have devoted a section to glue read that before you buy. This way you are armed with knowledge.

Most manufacturers suggest keeping in a cool dark cupboard not in the refrigerator

EYEBROW EXTENSIONS INFO

Indications for Eyebrow Extensions are perfect for anyone wanting fuller, or groomed eyebrows. Eyebrow extensions can be a life-changer for those who cannot grow full brows due to a variety of conditions, including: Over tweezing, or waxing through the years, scarring, hypothyroidism, alopecia, chemotherapy or aging.

EYEBROW EXTENSION APPLICATION

Eyebrow extensions are applied individually to existing eyebrow hairs, or directly onto the skin, giving client's full, beautifully shaped eyebrows.

NOTE: Eyebrow extensions can last up to three weeks when cared for properly.

SUPPLIES NEEDED:

Eyebrow extensions come in two diameters. .07mm, and .10mm, with .10mm being the diameter of choice. Brow extensions are typically straight with a very slight curve to them.

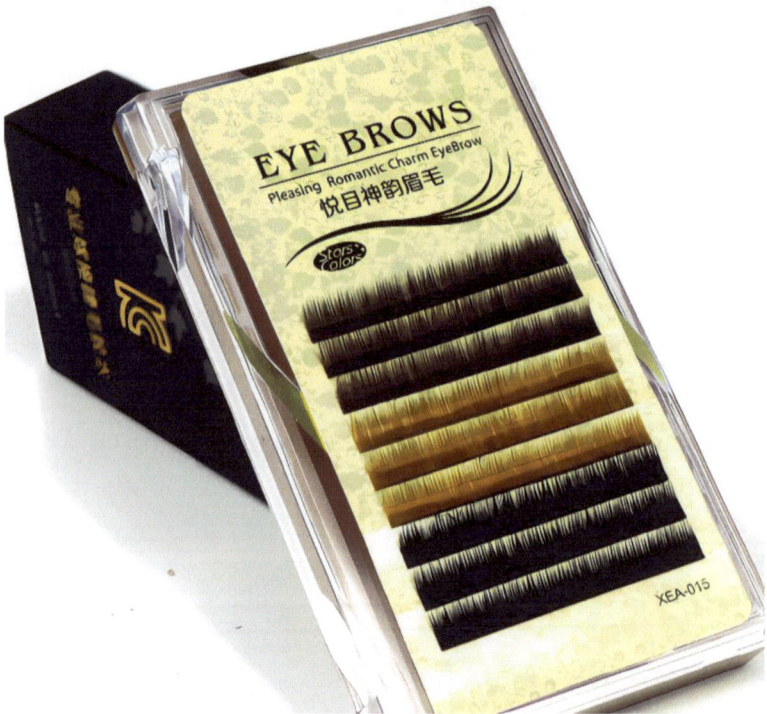

These are available on eBay Chocolate brown is the most used colour.

They come in multiple colours, including all variations of browns, from light to dark, auburn and black.

Care more so the client sings your praises.   Page | 2

I like this companies honesty. They say in their description not to get the glue on the skin.

Eyebrow adhesive is clear, low-fume, and most businesses say it is formulated to use on the skin. Unless they can back up that statement with Government documentation, you must ignore their statement.
I use my eyelash glue and avoid skin contact by folding each eyebrow hair up with a toothpick.

Straight tweezers are used to apply the extensions individually to the existing eyebrows.

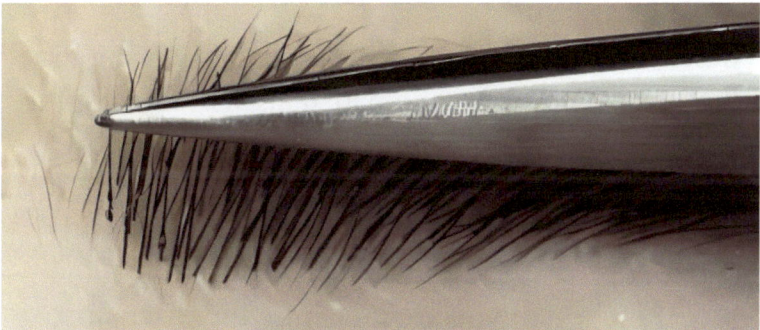

Isolate the hairs with tweezers. Note this student has done an amazing job of positioning the hairs but the glue is noticeable. View next enlarged photo.

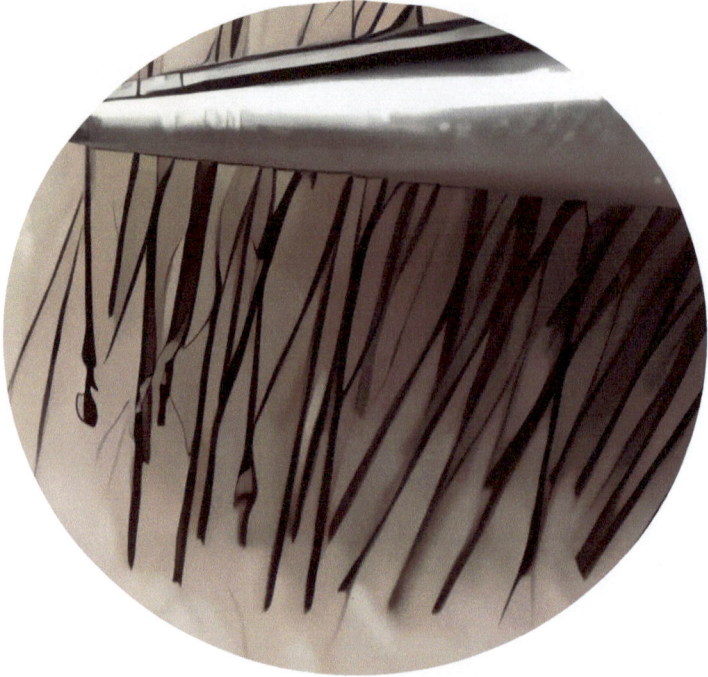

To avoid this situation - wipe the hair after you dip it in the glue on your jade pad. This will remove the excess glue before you attach the extension to the natural hair.

Use the air blower to dry the glue before releasing the tweezers that are holding the natural brow hair away from where you are attaching the extension.

Disposable mascara wands are used to groom and style the brows during the extension process.

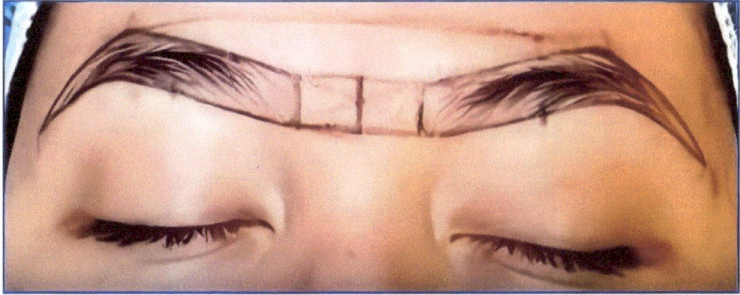

Use the provided diagram to create the perfect shape for every client. Before you begin the eyebrow extension process, use a white eyeliner pencil to mark and create a shape for your client. I used a dark pencil in this diagram so you could see the lines better.

As individuals everyones hair grows in different ways. Pay attention to this fact and think about where you are going to attach each hair. When trimming long hair consider clients bald patches. Some long hair should not be cut as it will expose a bald patch.

Brush their eyebrow hairs in a few different directions before trimming. Only trim after a full inspection.

Treat this application of eyebrow extensions as you would eyelash extensions and keep the glue away from the skin.

Each extension should be dried with the pump dryer.

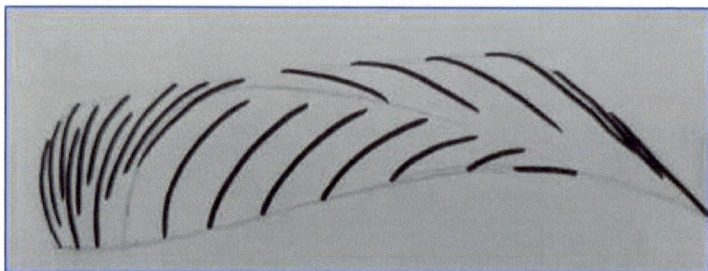

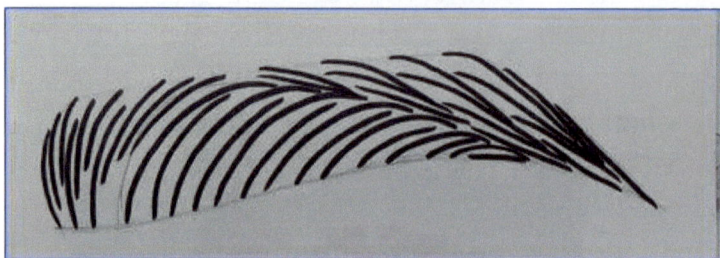

Always follow the way the natural hairs grow.

You can attach more than one extension to a natural eyebrow hair. You can also use a bridging hair that you can attach other extensions too.

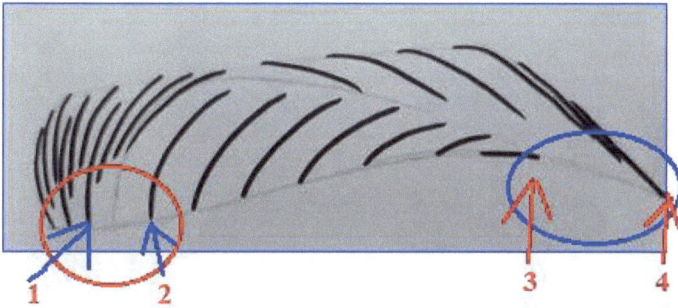

Bridge the gap with an extension

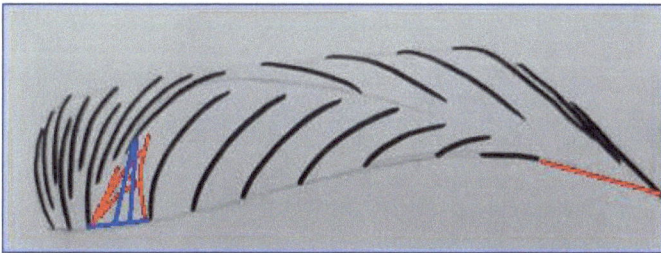

When their eyebrows have gaps you need to bridge the gap with an extension attached to the natural hair each side of the gap. Then add extensions to the bridging hair.

You can also add several extensions to the hair each side of the gap.

Broken Eyebrow — **A.**

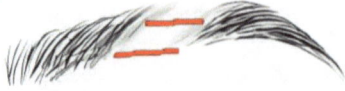

Attach Bridging Extensions

Short Eyebrow — **B.** 1. 2. 3.

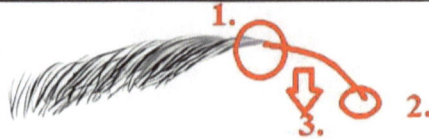

Attach Extensions to Skin

Shallow Eyebrow — **C.**

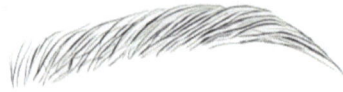

A. Where there is a gap attach an extension to the hair each side of the gap then add extensions to the bridging hair.

B. Attach an extension to the top of the last hair then glue the extension to the skin to form the end point. Next attach the extensions to the hair between points 1. and 2. In a downward position. Glue should not touch the skin but if attaching hair each side f the gap does not help you will need to attach to the bear skin. They will not last as long as attaching to a hair. Be sure you have done a patch test to assure yourself the client are not allergic to the glue.

C. Is a normal type of eyebrow that needs infills attached to the normal eyebrow hairs. Do so in the direction of the normal growth.

As I have explained, glue is not a product that should be attached to the skin. However, unless the client can afford the time and money to have transplants - you will need to attach extensions to the skin. Do so only after a patch test has been found - to not cause any skin irritations.

1. Begin your shape by taking the white pencil, or an orangewood stick and laying it vertically (straight up and down) at the outside corner of the nose.

2. Next, holding the pencil on the corner of the nose, angle it vertically so that it brushes past the outside corner of the pupil. Mark this area on top of your eyebrow. This should be the highest point of your eyebrow arch.

3. Lastly, with your pencil still on the corner of the nose, angle it vertically so that it brushes the outside corner of the eye. Mark this area of the eyebrow.

This is where your eyebrow should end. Using these marks as a guideline, create an eyebrow design. Determine where you need to remove hair or add your extensions.

 This is where your eyebrow should start. Mark this area with a white pencil.

However, you need to consider the width of their nose. For clients with a wide nose I prefer to use the A,B,C,D method.

EYEBROWS START AND END.

If you can never figure out where your eyebrows should start and where they should end. You probably don't have the right eyebrow shape for your face, and that is easily fixed with waxing and tinting.

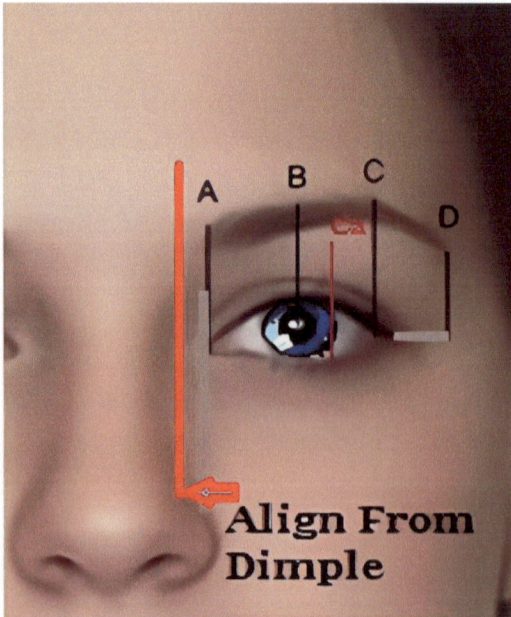

Align From Dimple

A. Will always start in line with either:- the outer edge of the nose or if you have a wide nose, start the line from the dimple in your nose. On some people with a narrow nose and bridge, the start point will need to be in line with the tear duct of the inner eye.

B. The eyebrow should have slightly tapered as you reach the B mark, which is the centre of your eye pupil.

C. Position "C: is for a peaked type of arch. The peak should be almost at the end of the eyelid outer corner. A peaked brow gives the illusion of a wider face and suits thin people. . For a plump wider face move the peak back to the "a" position.

D. The end of the brow should be a thumb space away from the outer corner of the eyelid or half the width of your nose.

Ca. A curved arch should be lined up to start at the end of the pupil. Be sure the client is looking straight ahead.

The client should lay in the beauty slant position so you are sitting well above her face.

TINTING THE EYEBROWS:

I like to always finish my eyebrow extensions with a good brow tint. You must use a brow tint specifically formulated for the area. Brow tints come in many colours.

However, this cannot be done successfully on the same day as the eyebrow extensions. Make a separate appointed time for the client to return after 24 to 48 hours. The glue takes at least 24 hours to cure/set.

Try to match the colour of the brow to the extensions as closely as possible. Tint can stain the delicate skin of the eye area and brows. Use this to your advantage.

Apply the tint perfectly with a small makeup brush. Apply it in your mapped areas and apply it cleanly in your desired end shape.

Process and remove according to manufacturer's recommendations.

SHAPING THE EYEBROWS:

Using a mascara wand and small manicure scissors, brush the eyebrows straight up and trim the excess hair, leaving a clean, groomed line. *Trim only after conducting a full inspection of their brows. Long hair often is hiding a bald patch.*

REMOVING EYEBROW EXTENSIONS:

Let the remover sit for approximately 10 minutes. You may have to reapply the remover, keeping it moist and active. Using two cotton swabs, brow comb and gel remover. Apply remover using a stroking motion from the base of the extensions, to the tips. Work the extensions free using a disposable mascara wand and damp gauze. Rinse and cleanse the eyebrows with damp gauze or cotton pads.

OTHER BOOKS BY

BEAUTY SCHOOL BOOKS

In 1995 I started writing training manuals for other companies. Prior to that, I had a protocol book in each of my salons for the staff. I am not a trained author nor claim to be a great writer but I am good at training. All too often when I gave young ladies the opportunity to do their workplace training at my salons I noticed, how raw they were. It is impossible for them to remember all they have been shown at college. I realized they needed to be reminded about the finer points on each module and that is how my procedures manuals evolved. On each procedure I had a page for the room setup, client comfort, Tray setup procedures and Procedure step by step instructions.

I have now added those note to what I call my "Beauty School Books Training Manuals" I always said one day I would write books for the industry and here they are:-

Aromatherapy Know How
This is a book that is very easy to follow with instructions on how to use essential oils correctly. It also contains an A-Z list of ailments and what oils to heal that ailment.

The Antique Healer

This book is jam packed with old wives tales, folklore medications and my favorite cures handed down to me via my grandparents and my mum. It also covers all my favorite essential oils their use and healing powers. With an A-Z list of ailments and cures for each ailment. This book has been in the making in my spare time for the past 22 years. I hope to release it by December 2015.

Spiritual Affirmations

Daily verses to keep you thinking in a wonderfully peaceful positively happy state of mind. Some verses have been composed by the author and other verses are by the great minds of yesteryear.

Life Your Life To The Next Level

Loaded with verses and affirmation, ideas on how to laugh and adjust to badly behaved friends and family.

Dogs DIY Medications.

There are many times you will not be able to afford a vet and sometimes when you cannot get to a veterinary clinic. This book will assist you where and when possible to heal your dog in those situation.

Natural Skincare Know How

For Acne, Acne Scars & Aging Skin. Skincare recipes that you can make at home. They have far better healing properties than store bought products. I have used these skincare products in my salons for over 50 years with amazing results.

Blossom Up Your Mind

A great book to keep your mind - in a healthy happy state.

Organic Cancer Cure.

Eyebrow Extension Training

This is what worked for my mum. It might work for you or someone you love.

How To Training Manuals.

Body Piercing Basics
All the main points on body piercing. Correct tray set up and procedures.

Anatomy For Body Piercers
All Body Piercers should understand the body and how it works this is a wonderful tool for any Body Piercer.

Eyelash Eyebrow Extension Training
Step by step instructions with video tutorials.

Create Eyebrows To Suit Face Shapes.
Step by step instructions with video tutorials on eyebrow shaping, eyelash and brow tinting.

Design & Perform Cosmetic Tattooing/Micro-pigmentation
A step by step training manual. You could actually teach yourself the trade. The books were tested on students that either live in remote areas and students wanting to learn from home the feedback from them has been very positive.

Hair Extensions Training Manual
Learn to create hair wefts, weaves, braids, wax in, and clip in Hair Extensions. There are videos to watch in the eBook.

Supernatural Books:-

Folklore & Spells

Learn More to Earn More

A great book on how to do some positive affirmations also called spells.

Tarot Scrolls
Ask a question open a page and an inspiring answer will be there for you to read.

Numerology Folklore
Numerology basics guide you through your birth force vibrations and your seasons of life. It is a short to the point book. Work out who you are and what you should be doing with your career in a heartbeat.

Children's Books:-

Mark Antony Is Born
A wonderful story, about a puppy born on a boat. His white, cute and fluffy. True storey with a dash of magic added.

Mark Antony Marries Lizy
Loaded with photos of all the dogs and the new born puppies. A true story with a dash of fantasy added.

By Robyn Ji Smith
Design & Perform Cosmetic Tattooing,
Micropigmentation: Follows International Training Standards Sibbsks504a (Beauty School Books)

Alluring Study Of Aromatherapy -For Healers &
Perfumers: Follows International Standards For Applying Aromatic Plants SIBBBOS505A (Beauty Pathways Elective Studies 3)

DIY Chakra Balancing: The Art of Connecting To Your Higher Self (New Age by Beauty School Books)Part of: New Age by Beauty School Books Robyn Ji Smith

Chakra Balancing version 2 Robyn Ji Smith

Learn Perfume Creating - With Natures Gifts: Organic and Alcohol Perfumes Edition 2 (Beauty School Books Training Manuals (For Beauty Pathways Academy) by Robyn ji Smith

Learn Perfume Creating -With Natures Gifts: Organic & Synthetic Edition 4 (Beauty Pathways Academy) by Robyn Ji-Smith

Learn Reiki Energy Healing version 2 Robyn Ji Smith

Learn Reiki & Chakra Balancing by Robyn Ji Smith

Got It: Inner Peace (Beauty Pathways Academy) **by Robyn Ji-Smith**
Sustaining A Positively Happy Mind
Diaries
Mindfulness and Gratefulness Diary: Edition 3 with Meditation
Diary Moon Moods Gratitude and Affirmations.
Gratitude and Gratefulness Diary

Blood Pressure And Heat Beat Log book

Our YouTube Channel.
https://www.youtube.com/channel/UCbH-MBFfJDSlBqgnRzZ06hQ
Reiki Video 1
https://www.youtube.com/watch?v=m8E5akEl2ho
https://www.youtube.com/watch?v=m8E5akEl2ho
Learn Perfume Creating Video 2
https://www.youtube.com/watch?v=3m_FSsQqWfQ

Care more so the client sings your praises.

Learning to create Organic Perfumes Video 1
https://www.youtube.com/watch?v=oKDUNYbuWmg&t=11
65s
Blending Essential Oils for lotions Video 2
https://www.youtube.com/watch?v=kVnkQv0kdOI&t=15
89s
Learn Body Piercing
https://www.youtube.com/watch?v=Bk3qOFvSa7w&t=10
s
Learn Cosmetic Tattooing
https://www.youtube.com/watch?v=2bAuFf6D1OQ&t=14
s
https://www.youtube.com/watch?v=iVFutf2sKP4&t=78s
https://www.youtube.com/channel/UCbH-
MBFfJDSlBqgnRzZ06hQ
https://www.youtube.com/watch?v=O8YqQiwwVHM&t=9s

You may contact the Author at
https://www.facebook.com/AromatherapyAndBeautySchool
Books
Email **mailto:beautyschoolbooks@gmail.com**
My Blog Page
Blog - Beauty School Books
https://beautyschoolbooks.com.au/blogs-on-natural-healings/.

Contact Robyn at mailto:beautyschoolbooks@gmail.com
http://www.beautyschoolbooks.com.au
http://www.thatsgreat.co
Join me on face book.
https://www.facebook.com/groups/FolkloreHealings/

I am in my 70s now so while I am alive and kicking I am
here to help. I am in no way an author trained to write.
However, I am good at training and know my trade. I am
here to help, so while I am still alive please feel free to ask

me questions via email. There is no charge for email questions.

Good luck everyone I pray this manual will assist you to flutter up with great looking lashes. I am only ever an email away from you if you are cross examining yourself or any information you have read.

It is hard to give you everything I think you need to know to become a great Beauty Therapist. Each of my Beauty School Books has its main topic and the title of each book contains hopefully all you need to know about that subject. I often add extracts from some of my other books as it seems relevant at the time of written for you.

I would like to take this opportunity to tell you how smart you are. Anyone that takes time to read all they can find on any given subject is a blessing to our trade.
You are a play safe individual.

Congratulations & My Blessing

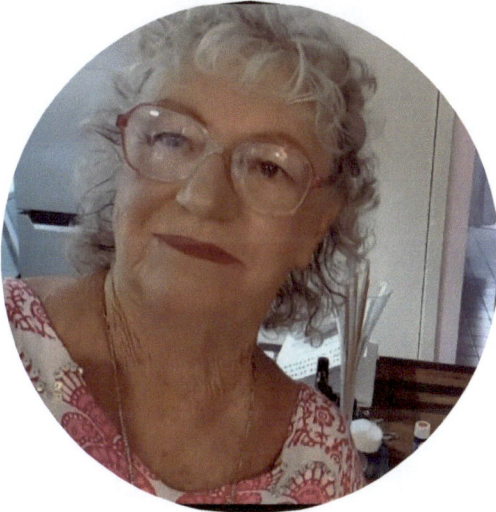

From Robyn X

If you live in Australia on the Gold Coast come and join my free Reiki group.

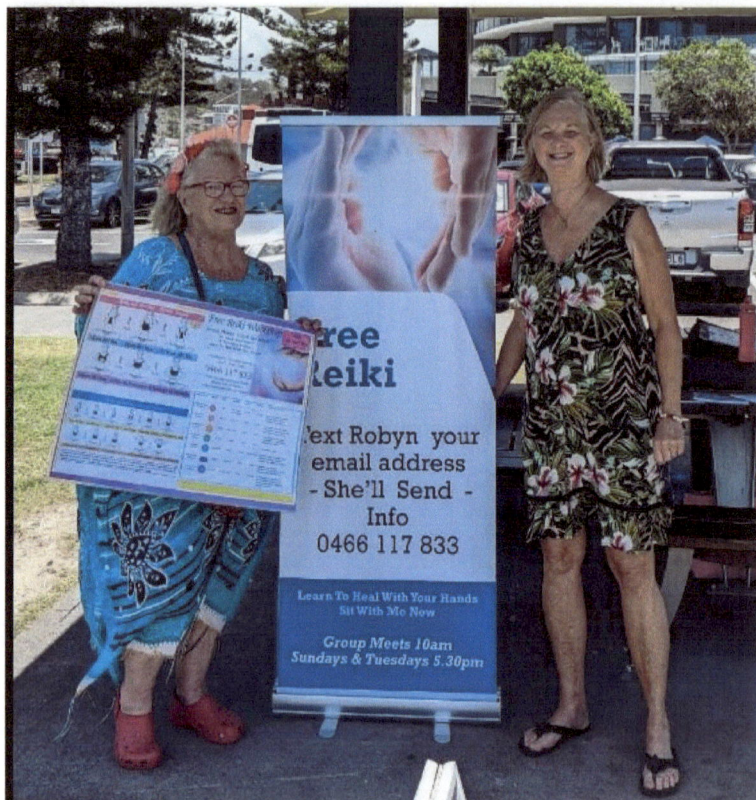